Periodontitis

Periodontitis

From Dysbiotic Microbial Immune Response to Systemic Inflammation

Editor

Anders Johansson

MDPI • Basel • Beijing • Wuhan • Barcelona • Belgrade • Manchester • Tokyo • Cluj • Tianjin

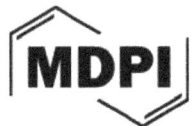

Editor
Anders Johansson
Umeå University
Sweden

Editorial Office
MDPI
St. Alban-Anlage 66
4052 Basel, Switzerland

This is a reprint of articles from the Special Issue published online in the open access journal *Journal of Clinical Medicine* (ISSN 2077-0383) (available at: https://www.mdpi.com/journal/jcm/special_issues/Periodontitis_Immune).

For citation purposes, cite each article independently as indicated on the article page online and as indicated below:

LastName, A.A.; LastName, B.B.; LastName, C.C. Article Title. *Journal Name* **Year**, *Article Number*, Page Range.

ISBN 978-3-03943-507-4 (Hbk)
ISBN 978-3-03943-508-1 (PDF)

© 2020 by the authors. Articles in this book are Open Access and distributed under the Creative Commons Attribution (CC BY) license, which allows users to download, copy and build upon published articles, as long as the author and publisher are properly credited, which ensures maximum dissemination and a wider impact of our publications.

The book as a whole is distributed by MDPI under the terms and conditions of the Creative Commons license CC BY-NC-ND.

Contents

About the Editor vii

Jan Oscarsson and Anders Johansson
Comment from the Editor to the Special Issue: "Periodontitis: From Dysbiotic Microbial Immune Response to Systemic Inflammation"
Reprinted from: *Journal of Clinical Medicine* **2019**, *8*, 1706, doi:10.3390/jcm8101706 1

Nagihan Bostanci, Toshiharu Abe, Georgios N. Belibasakis and George Hajishengallis
TREM-1 Is Upregulated in Experimental Periodontitis, and Its Blockade Inhibits IL-17A and RANKL Expression and Suppresses Bone Loss
Reprinted from: *Journal of Clinical Medicine* **2019**, *8*, 1579, doi:10.3390/jcm8101579 5

Milla Pietiäinen, John M. Liljestrand, Ramin Akhi, Kåre Buhlin, Anders Johansson, Susanna Paju, Aino Salminen, Päivi Mäntylä, Juha Sinisalo, Leo Tjäderhane, Sohvi Hörkkö and Pirkko J. Pussinen
Saliva and Serum Immune Responses in Apical Periodontitis
Reprinted from: *Journal of Clinical Medicine* **2019**, *8*, 889, doi:10.3390/jcm8060889 19

Gunnar Dahlen, Amina Basic and Johan Bylund
Importance of Virulence Factors for the Persistence of Oral Bacteria in the Inflamed Gingival Crevice and in the Pathogenesis of Periodontal Disease
Reprinted from: *Journal of Clinical Medicine* **2019**, *8*, 1339, doi:10.3390/jcm8091339 35

Eduardo Gómez-Bañuelos, Amarshi Mukherjee, Erika Darrah and Felipe Andrade
Rheumatoid Arthritis-Associated Mechanisms of *Porphyromonas gingivalis* and *Aggregatibacter actinomycetemcomitans*
Reprinted from: *Journal of Clinical Medicine* **2019**, *8*, 1309, doi:10.3390/jcm8091309 55

Eija Könönen, Mervi Gursoy and Ulvi Kahraman Gursoy
Periodontitis: A Multifaceted Disease of Tooth-Supporting Tissues
Reprinted from: *Journal of Clinical Medicine* **2019**, *8*, 1135, doi:10.3390/jcm8081135 79

Melissa M. Grant and Daniel Jönsson
Next Generation Sequencing Discoveries of the Nitrate-Responsive Oral Microbiome and Its Effect on Vascular Responses
Reprinted from: *Journal of Clinical Medicine* **2019**, *8*, 1110, doi:10.3390/jcm8081110 91

Jan Oscarsson, Rolf Claesson, Mark Lindholm, Carola Höglund Åberg and Anders Johansson
Tools of *Aggregatibacter actinomycetemcomitans* to Evade the Host Response
Reprinted from: *Journal of Clinical Medicine* **2019**, *8*, 1079, doi:10.3390/jcm8071079 101

About the Editor

Anders Johansson, PhD, Associate Professor. Dr. Johansson is a docent in experimental periodontology and has been active for several decades at Umeå University, focusing on the major research topics of the interactions between A. actinomycetemcomitans and leukocytes. Dr. Johansson and co-workers have discovered active processes in leukocytes that have been induced by leukotoxin, like neutrophil degranulation and inflammasome activation in macrophages. The research has also involved clinical studies that contributed to clarifying the role of enhanced leukotoxin production for disease progression.

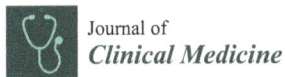

Editorial

Comment from the Editor to the Special Issue: "Periodontitis: From Dysbiotic Microbial Immune Response to Systemic Inflammation"

Jan Oscarsson and Anders Johansson *

Department of Odontology, Umeå University, S-901 87 Umeå, Sweden; jan.oscarsson@umu.se
* Correspondence: anders.p.johansson@umu.se; Tel.: +46-90-7856291

Received: 14 October 2019; Accepted: 15 October 2019; Published: 16 October 2019

Abstract: The human oral cavity contains a large number of different microbial habitats. When microbes from the oral indigenous flora colonize the interspace between the tooth and the connective tissue, they induce an inflammatory response. If the microbes are in sufficient numbers, and release components that cause an imbalance in the host inflammatory response, degenerative processes in the surrounding tissues are induced, ultimately resulting in periodontal disease. The disease progress depends on bacterial load, the composition of the microbial community, and host genetic factors. The two most studied periodontal pathogens, *Porphyromonas gingivalis* and *Aggregatibacter actinomycetemcomitans* express virulence factors, including proteases and exotoxins. Periodontal infections are also linked to the risk pattern of several systemic diseases. We would like to shed light on the mechanisms behind periodontitis and the associations of periodontal infections with systemic inflammation. Seven articles are included in this Special Issue and cover several pathogenic processes in the periodontal infection with capacity to cause imbalance in the host response. Highlights from each of the published papers are summarized and discussed below.

Keywords: periodontitis; cardiovascular diseases; rheumatoid arthritis; *Porphyromonas gingivalis*; *Aggregatibacter actinomycetemcomitans*; inflammatory response

---

This Special Issue discusses the factors that induce a dysbiotic microbial periodontal immune response in periodontitis, which might result in a systemic inflammation. Könönen and co-workers [1] define periodontitis as an infection-driven inflammatory disease, by which the composition of the microbial biofilms play a significant role. Moreover, genetics and environmental or behavioral factors are involved in the development of the disease and its progression. The authors conclude that periodontal disease is multifactorial and the imbalance between tissue loss and gain can occur, due to various reasons, including aggressive infection, uncontrolled chronic inflammation, weakened healing, or all of the above simultaneously. Thus, successful disease management requires an understanding of the different elements of the disease at the individual level, and the design of personalized treatment modalities, including immunotherapies and modulators of inflammation.

In the second paper, Dahlén et al. [2] emphasize that the role of the classic, putative periodontal pathogens in the disease is still unclear, and the infectious nature of periodontitis today is in question. However, there is an enormous complexity and variability that takes place, both within the dental biofilm communities and in the inflammatory response, which makes it challenging to disclose the actual roles of specific microorganisms in periodontitis. Inflammation in the gingiva (gingivitis) is a normal host tissue response, induced by commensal microorganisms and their released products (metabolites, endotoxins). The infectious nature of the microbes, and the extent to which the specific virulence factors induce a dysbiotic host response leading to an impaired tissue repair, remain unclear. Most of the factors discussed in terms of virulence (proteases, LPS, invasive ability, fimbriae, capsule, and leukotoxin), among the microorganisms that are commonly associated with periodontitis, should rather be termed microbial survival factors. One exception is the leukotoxin produced by *Aggregatibacter actinomycetemcomitans*, which highly leukotoxic genotype (JP2) best fulfils the designation of a periodontal pathogen in the human oral microbiota. Presence of the JP2 genotype in periodontally healthy adolescents has previously been shown to be a strong risk marker for a future development of periodontal attachment loss.

A. actinomycetemcomitans is a facultative anaerobic Gram-negative bacterium that induces cellular and molecular mechanisms, and is associated with the pathogenesis of periodontitis. This bacterium is present in the oral cavity of a large proportion of the human population. However, its association to disease is mainly limited to young carriers. In their review, Oscarsson and co-workers [3] discuss virulence mechanisms that enable *A. actinomycetemcomitans* to evade the host response. These properties include invasiveness, secretion of exotoxins, serum resistance, and release of outer membrane vesicles. It is today hypothesized that the virulence characteristics of *A. actinomycetemcomitans* allow this organism to induce an immune subversion that tips the balance from homeostasis over to disease in oral and/or extra-oral sites. Hence, in order to prohibit the negative systemic consequences that are associated with periodontitis, successful treatment in an early phase of the disease is fundamental. The development of specific diagnostic tools for the assessment of periodontal pathogens and inflammatory components in the saliva of young individuals might make it possible to prevent the disease before its onset.

Antigens, released from the periodontal bacteria, activate both, a local and systemic immune response. These responses normally prevents microbial invasion deeper into the tissues surrounding the teeth, or into circulation. The work by Pietiäinen and collaborators [4] focuses on the immune response against bacteria occurring in apical periodontitis, an inflammatory disease that affects the tissues surrounding the apex of the tooth, which is initially triggered by oral pathogens infecting the root canals. The study investigated serum and saliva antibodies against several oral pathogens associated with apical periodontitis, and the role of cross-reactive antibodies in the disease. The authors concluded that this form of periodontitis associates with adaptive immune responses against both bacterial- and host-derived epitopes, in line with other forms of periodontitis. In addition, their results indicate that salivary immunoglobulins could be useful biomarkers in oral infections, including apical periodontitis, a putative risk factor for systemic diseases.

A number of host-derived risk marker candidates, associated with periodontal inflammation, have been the focus of many different experimental studies. The triggering receptor, that is expressed on myeloid cells-1 (TREM-1), a modifier of local and systemic inflammation, has been studied by Bostanci and co-workers [5]. Bacterial infections can upregulate the membrane-bound and soluble forms of TREM-1, which in turn amplifies inflammation. The blockade of TREM-1 engagement by either soluble forms of TREM-1 or synthetic peptides reduces the hyper-inflammatory responses and morbidity. The result obtained in the present study demonstrated the involvement of TREM-1 in alveolar bone resorption during the course of experimental periodontitis in mice. TREM-1 reduced the RANKL/OPG osteoclastogenic ratio, presumably via the inhibition of IL-17. The authors suggest that a previously unidentified TREM-1-driven axis for inflammatory bone loss could be targeted via small-molecule antagonists for therapeutic intervention in human periodontitis.

An association between cardiovascular diseases (CVD) and periodontitis has been established over the past several decades. Grant and Jönsson [6] focus their review on the association between the oral microbiota and the most well-established mechanistic pathway by which the oral microbiota may modify CVD, namely via the nitric oxide (NO) synthesis pathway. Next generation sequencing has been used over the past two decades to gain deeper insight into the microbes involved, their location, and the effect of their removal from the oral cavity. Overall, these studies have demonstrated that there are nitrate and nitrite-reducing bacteria found in the mouth, and that their removal causes systemic effects, i.e., through a temporary increase in blood pressure. The authors have highlighted the role of the oral microbiota in the conversion of nitrate to nitrite and its importance to systemic balance.

A deeper understanding of the role of oral microbiota will allow future interventions to proceed, including personalized medicine approaches, and potentially reduce the use of antimicrobials.

Another systemic disease associated with periodontitis is rheumatoid arthritis (RA). This is an autoimmune disease of unknown etiology, characterized by immune-mediated damage of synovial joints and antibodies to citrullinated antigens. Gómez-Bañuelos and co-workers [7] discussed the clinical and mechanistic evidence concerning the role of the common periodontal pathogens *A. actinomycetemcomitans* and *Porphyromonas gingivalis* in RA pathogenesis. Both these pathobionts exhibit virulence mechanisms that promote citrullination of proteins, which indicate a possible involvement in the formation of the RA-associated autoantibodies against citrullinated antigens. For example, *P. gingivalis* produces a peptidylarginine deaminase that converts arginine to citrulline, and the *A. actinomycetemcomitans* leukotoxin activates neutrophil degranulation, which results in release of extracellular net-like structures that contains citrullinated proteins. The authors concluded that these oral pathobionts, together, give an opportunity to understand whether bacterial-associated citrullination is a mechanism involved in RA pathogenesis. These discoveries have the potential to be used in the implementation of future preventive interventions in RA.

We can conclude that the articles in this Special Issue give a comprehensive overview of the complex interplay between the oral microbiota and the host response, which can induce the degenerative processes in the tooth supporting tissues, ultimately resulting in periodontitis. Increased knowledge about these biological processes will contribute to the development of improved preventive and treatment strategies for periodontal disease. New biomarker candidates, that are the potential targets for therapeutic strategies, are continuously discovered and could make personalized dentistry into a reality in the future.

Acknowledgments: We acknowledge all the authors of the seven papers for their contribution, which made this Special Issue a valuable and comprehensive work.

Conflicts of Interest: The authors declare no conflict of interest.

References

1. Könönen, E.; Gursoy, M.; Gursoy, U.K. Periodontitis: A multifaceted disease of tooth-supporting tissues. *J. Clin. Med.* **2019**, *8*, 1135. [CrossRef] [PubMed]
2. Dahlen, G.; Basic, A.; Bylund, J. Importance of virulence factors for the persistence of oral bacteria in the inflamed gingival crevice and in the pathogenesis of periodontal disease. *J. Clin. Med.* **2019**, *8*, 1339. [CrossRef] [PubMed]
3. Oscarsson, J.; Claesson, R.; Lindholm, M.; Höglund Åberg, C.; Johansson, A. Tools of *Aggregatibacter actinomycetemcomitans* to evade the host response. *J. Clin. Med.* **2019**, *8*, 1079. [CrossRef] [PubMed]
4. Pietiäinen, M.; Liljestrand, J.M.; Akhi, R.; Buhlin, K.; Johansson, A.; Paju, S.; Salminen, A.; Mäntyla, P.; Sinisalo, J.; Tjäderhane, L.; et al. Saliva and serum immune responses in apical periodontitis. *J. Clin. Med.* **2019**, *8*, 889. [CrossRef] [PubMed]
5. Bostanci, N.; Abe, T.; Belibasakis, G.N.; Hajishengallis, G. TREM-1 is upregulated in experimental periodontitis, and its blockade inhibits IL-17A and RANKL expression and suppresses bone loss. *J. Clin. Med.* **2019**, *8*, 1579. [CrossRef] [PubMed]
6. Grant, M.M.; Jönsson, D. Next generation sequencing discoveries of the nitrate-responsive oral microbiome and its effect on vascular responses. *J. Clin. Med.* **2019**, *8*, 1110. [CrossRef] [PubMed]
7. Gomez-Banuelos, E.; Mukherjee, A.; Darrah, E.; Andrade, F. Rheumatoid arthritis-associated mechanisms of *Porphyromonas gingivalis* and *Aggregatibacter actinomycetemcomitans*. *J. Clin. Med.* **2019**, *8*, 1309. [CrossRef] [PubMed]

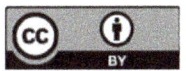

© 2019 by the authors. Licensee MDPI, Basel, Switzerland. This article is an open access article distributed under the terms and conditions of the Creative Commons Attribution (CC BY) license (http://creativecommons.org/licenses/by/4.0/).

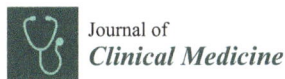

Article

TREM-1 Is Upregulated in Experimental Periodontitis, and Its Blockade Inhibits IL-17A and RANKL Expression and Suppresses Bone Loss

Nagihan Bostanci [1,2,*], Toshiharu Abe [3], Georgios N. Belibasakis [1,2] and George Hajishengallis [3]

1. Division of Oral Diseases, Department of Dental Medicine, Karolinska Institutet, 14104 Huddinge, Sweden; george.belibasakis@ki.se
2. Center of Dental Medicine, University of Zürich, 8032 Zürich, Switzerland
3. Department of Basic and Translational Sciences, School of Dental Medicine, University of Pennsylvania, Philadelphia, PA 19104, USA; toshiharu@ikeshita-abeshika.com (T.A.); geoh@upenn.edu (G.H.)
* Correspondence: nagihan.bostanci@ki.se

Received: 10 September 2019; Accepted: 24 September 2019; Published: 1 October 2019

Abstract: Aim: Triggering receptor expressed on myeloid cells-1 (TREM-1) is a modifier of local and systemic inflammation. There is clinical evidence implicating TREM-1 in the pathogenesis of periodontitis. However, a cause-and-effect relationship has yet to be demonstrated, as is the underlying mechanism. The aim of this study was to elucidate the role of TREM-1 using the murine ligature-induced periodontitis model. Methods: A synthetic antagonistic LP17 peptide or sham control was microinjected locally into the palatal gingiva of the ligated molar teeth. Results: Mice treated with the LP17 inhibitor developed significantly less bone loss as compared to sham-treated mice, although there were no differences in total bacterial load on the ligatures. To elucidate the impact of LP17 on the host response, we analyzed the expression of a number of immune-modulating genes. The LP17 peptide altered the expression of 27/92 genes ≥ two-fold, but only interleukin (IL)-17A was significantly downregulated (4.9-fold). Importantly, LP17 also significantly downregulated the receptor activator of nuclear factor kappa-B-ligand (RANKL) to osteoprotegerin (OPG) ratio that drives osteoclastic bone resorption in periodontitis. Conclusion: Our findings show for the first time that TREM-1 regulates the IL-17A-RANKL/OPG axis and bone loss in experimental periodontitis, and its therapeutic blockade may pave the way to a novel treatment for human periodontitis.

Keywords: TREM-1; periodontal disease; intervention; inflammation; LP17; IL-17; RANKL; OPG

1. Introduction

Periodontitis entails the destruction of the tooth-supporting (periodontal) tissues, as an outcome of their inflammatory response to the juxtaposed microbial biofilm forming on the tooth surface [1,2]. Although oral bacteria are essential for initiation of the disease, the resulting inflammation is what causes collateral damage to the tissues, which may eventually lead to tooth loss. The inflammatory mediators that lead to alveolar bone destruction form an intricate network [3,4], in which the receptor activator of NF-κB ligand (RANKL)/osteoprotegerin (OPG) system plays a crucial role as a terminal regulator of the resulting osteoclastogenesis and bone resorption [5,6]. Recently discovered host molecules, acting between the microbial challenge and the RANKL/OPG system, may lead to better understanding of the pathogenesis of periodontal disease and offer novel targets for therapeutic intervention.

Triggering receptor expressed on myeloid cells 1 (TREM-1), a member of the immunoglobulin superfamily, has been defined as a modifier of local and systemic inflammation, especially in response to bacterial infections [7–9]. Bacterial infection can upregulate the membrane-bound and soluble forms of TREM-1, which in turn amplifies inflammation. This is a particularly crucial response associated with systemic sepsis [10,11]. Blockade of TREM-1 engagement by either soluble forms of TREM-1 or synthetic peptides thereof reduces hyper-inflammatory responses and morbidity [12]. In a TREM-1 knock-out mouse model of viral or parasitic infection, it was demonstrated that the lack of TREM-1 signaling mitigated the severity of inflammation and disease (as compared to the wild-type mice) without, however, affecting pathogen clearance [13]. The study by Weber et al. [13] suggested that TREM-1 regulates inflammation, and that its therapeutic targeting may be beneficial in infection-driven inflammatory diseases without compromising pathogen clearance.

There is also correlative evidence to suggest that TREM-1 might modify periodontal inflammation. Specifically, the presence or expression of TREM-1 is increased in saliva, serum [14,15], gingival crevicular fluid [16–18], and gingival tissues [19] of patients with periodontitis as compared to individuals with periodontal health. TREM-1 levels also positively correlate with the levels of putative periodontal pathogens present in subgingival biofilms or lysed gingival tissue [16,19]. In this respect, multispecies biofilms [19] or *Porphyromonas gingivalis* alone induce TREM-1 gene expression in monocytes [20], whereas sub-antimicrobial doses of doxycycline can abolish this upregulatory effect [21].

The studies discussed above collectively suggest that TREM-1 expression is upregulated in periodontitis as a result of microbial stimulation. However, there are as-yet no interventional studies in preclinical models to conclusively demonstrate TREM-1 involvement in periodontitis. Hence, this in vivo study in a validated model of murine ligature-induced periodontitis [22] was designed to investigate the effect of local TREM-1 inhibition on the induction of experimental periodontitis, as well as on the expression of inflammation- and osteoclastogenesis-associated molecules in the gingival tissue. Our results described below implicate for the first time TREM-1 in the pathogenesis of periodontitis in a preclinical model and suggest a novel therapeutic approach for the treatment of this oral inflammatory disease.

2. Materials and Methods

2.1. Ligature-Induced Periodontitis Model in Mice

The well-established ligature-induced periodontitis model in specific pathogen-free C57BL/6 mice was used as described earlier [22]. All animal procedures were performed according to protocols approved by the Institutional Animal Care and Use Committee of the University of Pennsylvania, and adequate measures were taken to minimize pain or discomfort. To induce experimental periodontitis, a 5-0 silk ligature was tied around the maxillary left second molar for up to 8 days (n = 4–5 mice/group). The unligated contralateral molar in each mouse was used as baseline control (unligated control). A synthetic peptide derived from the extracellular domain of TREM-1 (LP17; LQVTDSGLYRCVIYHPP, Pepscan, Lelystad, Netherlands) was used as described earlier [7]. The LP17 blocking peptide is considered as a competitive antagonist of membrane-bound TREM-1 for its natural ligand, therefore acting as a decoy receptor for TREM signaling [23]. For the intervention experiments performed in this study, 5 µg of LP17 peptide or PBS were injected into the palatal gingiva of the ligated second maxillary molar 1 days before placing the ligature and every day thereafter until the day before sacrifice (day 5).

The measurements on the alveolar bone height were done on defleshed maxillae under a Nikon SMZ800 microscope (Nikon Instruments, Melville, NY, USA), and images of the maxillae were captured using a Nikon Digital Sight DS-U3 camera controller. The distance between the cemento-enamel junction (CEJ) and alveolar bone crest (ABC) was measured at six predetermined points on the ligated molar and adjacent regions using NIS Elements software (Nikon Instruments, Melville, NY, USA) [22]. To calculate bone loss, the six-site total CEJ–ABC distance for the ligated side of each mouse was subtracted from the six-site total CEJ–ABC distance of the contralateral unligated side. The results are presented in millimeters, and negative values indicate bone loss relative to the unligated control.

2.2. Bacterial Counts on Silk Sutures

The ligated silk sutures obtained from LP17-treated or PBS-treated mice at day 5 were collected (n = 5 mice/group). These were suspended individually in sterile PBS, and adherent bacteria were disassociated from the sutures via high-speed vortexing for 2 min. Serial dilutions of the samples were plated onto blood agar plates (BD Difco Laboratories, Detroit, MI, USA), and the plates were incubated anaerobically at 37 °C for 7 days. Results are reported as the mean number of colony forming units (CFUs) per millimeter length of silk suture ± the standard error of the mean (SEM). Anaerobic CFUs were preferred over aerobic ones because of the stronger etiological association of anaerobic organisms with periodontitis.

2.3. Antimicrobial Effects of the Synthetic Peptides in Vitro

A 6-species oral biofilm model was used to investigate the potential antimicrobial effects of LP17. The biofilm consisted of *Actinomyces oris* OMZ 745, *Veillonella dispar* OMZ 493 (ATCC 17748T), *Fusobacterium nucleatum* OMZ 598 (KP-F2), *Streptococcus mutans* OMZ 918 (UA159), *Streptococcus oralis* OMZ 607 (SK 248), and *Candida albicans* OMZ 110. In brief, biofilms were grown according to the standard protocol in 24-well cell culture plates on sintered hydroxyapatite (HA) discs, which were pre-conditioned for 4 h with pooled human saliva, for pellicle formation. Throughout the following experimentation period, the biofilms were grown in the presence of LP17 or 0.9% NaCl (sham control). After 5 days of biofilm growth under anaerobic conditions, the HA discs were vortexed vigorously for 1 min in 1 mL of 0.9% NaCl and then sonicated (Branson Sonic Power Company, Danbury, CT, USA) for 5 s to harvest the adherent biofilms. Then, to determine the total CFUs, the bacterial suspensions were serially diluted in 0.9% NaCl and 50 µL aliquots were plated on agar plates supplemented with 5% whole human blood at 37 °C for 72 h.

2.4. Quantitative TaqMan Real-Time PCR and TaqMan Array Analysis

The TaqMan Array 96-well Mouse Immune Response kit (Applied Biosystems) was used to assess the expression of 92 predetermined genes mediating the immune response and four endogenous control genes including *GAPDH, HPRT, GUSB and 18S RNA*. For this analysis, gingival tissues were collected at day 5 (n = 3 mice/group). Total RNA was extracted from these tissues by Qiagen Fibrous Tissue Extraction kit. According to the manufacturer's protocol, cDNA was mixed with 2× TaqMan Universal Master Mix and H_2O to a total volume of 2160 µL. Subsequently, 20 µL of the mixture was placed into each well of the PCR array. The three steps of the cycling program were 95 °C for 10 min for 1 cycle, then 95 °C for 15 s, and 60 °C for 1 min for 40 cycles, using a Step One Plus Real-Time PCR System (Applied Biosystems). In addition, the transcription levels of TREM-1, interleukin (IL)-1β, RANKL, OPG, COX-2, and IL-6 were assessed by individual TaqMan Gene Expression Assays (Applied Biosytems). For TaqMan qPCR analysis, mouse ACTB (β-actin) was used as an endogenous control.

2.5. Statistical Analysis

All statistical analyses were performed using Prism v.6.0 software (GraphPad Software, La Jolla, CA, USA). One-way ANOVA was used to determine differences between three or more groups, whereas an unpaired, two-tailed Student *t* test was used to determine the statistical significance of differences between two groups. Differences were considered significant at $p < 0.05$.

3. Results

3.1. Local Tissue Kinetics of TREM-1 Expression in Ligature-Induced Periodontitis

Using the ligature-induced murine periodontitis model, we first investigated the regulation of TREM-1 expression in the gingival tissue. TREM-1 gene expression was significantly upregulated at the ligated sites in a time-dependent manner, peaking at day 8 compared to the unligated control sites forming the baseline (Figure 1A). Compared to the unligated control sites, TREM-1 mRNA levels in the ligated sites were approximately 16-fold and 17-fold higher at day 5 and day 8, respectively ($p < 0.01$). Since TREM-1 activation is involved in the upregulation of a number of key proinflammatory cytokines [20], including IL-1β, which is crucial in periodontal pathogenesis, IL-1β gene expression levels were also assessed. A similar expression pattern was observed for IL-1β. In particular, compared to the baseline control, IL-1β gene expression at ligated sites was approximately 13-fold, 21-fold, and 27-fold higher at days 3, 5, and 8, respectively ($p < 0.01$) (Figure 1B).

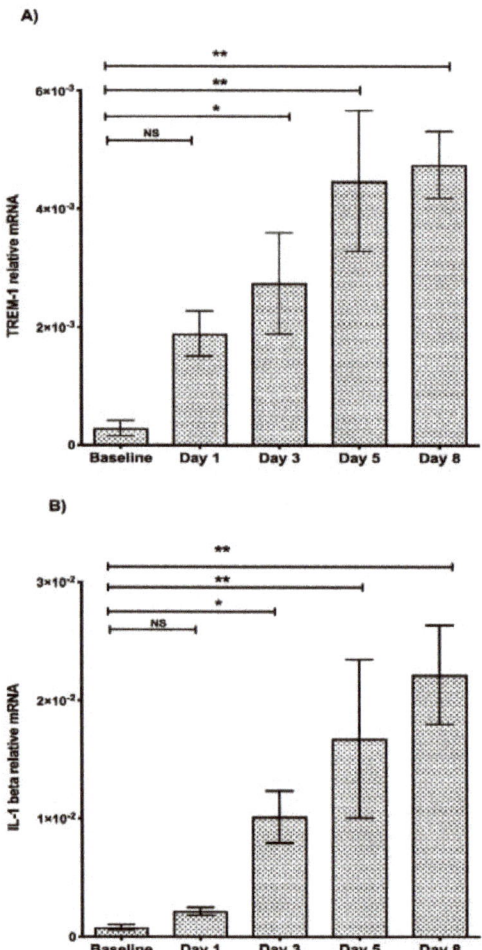

Figure 1. Kinetics of gingival tissue expression of TREM-1 and IL-1 beta in ligature-induced periodontitis. TREM-1 mRNA (**A**) and IL-1 beta mRNA (**B**) levels were examined in unligated control gingiva and ligature-induced periodontitis gingival tissues at 1 to 8 days. The gene expression levels were detected by TaqMan real-time qPCR and calibrated against the expression of housekeeping gene β-actin. Results are means ± SEM ($n = 4$ mice/group). * $p < 0.05$ and ** $p < 0.01$ between the indicated groups.

3.2. Role of TREM-1 in Alveolar Bone Loss

The kinetics of TREM-1 gene expression followed a pattern similar to those of ligature-induced bone loss seen in our previous publication [22]. To determine whether there was a cause-and-effect relationship between gingival TREM-1 expression and alveolar bone loss, we subjected groups of mice to ligature-induced periodontitis with local administration of the LP17 or with PBS sham control. Five days after placement of the ligatures, mice treated with LP17 developed significantly less alveolar bone loss as compared to the sham-treated mice ($p < 0.05$) (Figure 2A,B), indicating that TREM-1 signaling contributes to induction of alveolar bone loss.

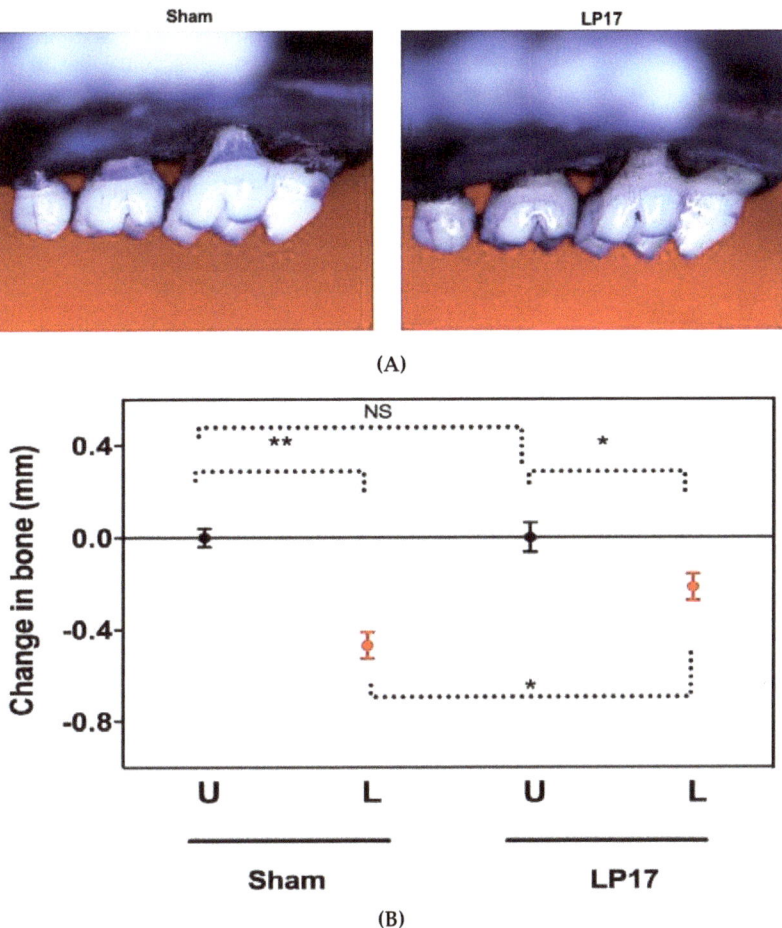

Figure 2. Inhibition of ligature-induced bone loss by LP17. Ligatures were placed on the left maxillary molars of C57BL/6 mice and then locally microinjected with 5 µg of TREM-1 blocking peptide (LP17) or with PBS sham 1 day before placing the ligature and every day thereafter until day 5. The distance between the cemento-enamel junction (CEJ) and alveolar bone crest (ABC) was measured at six predetermined points on the ligated side. Representative images of PBS sham- and LP17-treated maxillae exhibiting differential bone loss (**A**). To calculate bone loss, the six-site total CEJ–ABC distance for the ligated (L) side of each mouse was subtracted from the six-site total CEJ–ABC distance of the contralateral unligated (U) side. The results are presented in millimeters, and negative values indicate bone loss relative to the unligated control (**B**). Data are means ± SEM (n = 4–5 mice/group). * $p < 0.05$ and ** $p < 0.01$ between the indicated groups.

3.3. Investigation of Potential LP17 Antimicrobial Activity

To determine whether the protective effects of LP17 in ligature-induced periodontitis could, in part, be attributed to potential antimicrobial effects, we determined the microbial load of the treated mice from the above-described in vivo experiment (Figure 2). To this end, bacteria were extracted from the recovered ligatures (day 5) and cultivated anaerobically for 7 days on blood agar plates. To normalize the data, the counted CFUs were divided by the length of corresponding suture, and the results revealed that sutures from the LP17-treated mice yielded similar CFUs, as compared to the PBS sham-treated group ($p > 0.05$) (Figure 3A). Furthermore, the potential antimicrobial impact of LP17 was tested in vitro on a 6-species biofilm model for 5 days. A 1.3-fold reduction in total CFUs was observed, compared to the saline sham-treated group ($p > 0.05$). These results suggested that the LP17 peptide preferentially acted by regulating the host response rather than bacterial growth. Hence, we next investigated the host-modulating activity of LP17.

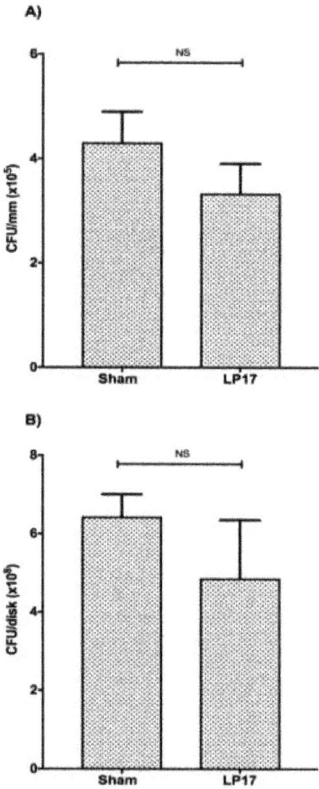

Figure 3. LP17 does not affect the microbial load in vivo. (**A**) Detached material from the recovered ligatures at day 5 from mice used in Figure 2 were cultivated anaerobically for 7 days on blood agar plates, followed by total colony forming unit (CFU) determination. To normalize the data, the counted CFUs were divided by the length of corresponding suture. Data are means ± SEM (n = 5 mice/group). NS: Not significant, $p > 0.05$. (**B**) LP17 does not affect the microbial load in vitro. The in vitro biofilms were grown in the presence of LP17 or 0.9% NaCl (sham). After 5 days of biofilm growth under anaerobic conditions, biofilm bacteria were harvested from the discs and cultivated anaerobically for 3 days on blood agar plates, followed by total CFU determination. The CFUs are given per hydroxyapatite (HA) disc. Data are means ± SEM (n = 3 disc /group). NS: Not significant, $p > 0.05$.

3.4. Modulation of Immunoregulatory Genes by TREM-1

To understand how TREM-1 signaling regulates the host periodontal response, the defleshed gingival tissues were analyzed for the expression of a number of immunoregulatory genes at day 5, by using a mouse immune response qPCR Array profiling for 92 individual genes (Table S1). Differential expression analysis was done by the following pair-wise comparisons: (a) unligated sites versus ligated sites and (b) PBS sham-treated ligated sites versus LP17-treated ligated sites. Although a basal expression level was detected for all studied genes at unligated control sites, a total of 38 genes were differentially transcribed by more than two-fold during the experimental infection period (Table S1). Among those, 27 genes were induced in the ligature-induced gingival sites, 7 of which reached statistical significance ($p < 0.05$). Another 11 genes were repressed more than two-fold, 7 of which also reached statistical significance ($p < 0.05$). The significantly upregulated genes were *IL-17A, IL-1β, CD80, CCR4, HMOX1, VEGFA,* and *CD68*, whereas the significantly downregulated ones were *SKI, SMAD 7, IL-7, NFATC 3, FAS, IL-15,* and *SMAD 3* (Figure 4A).

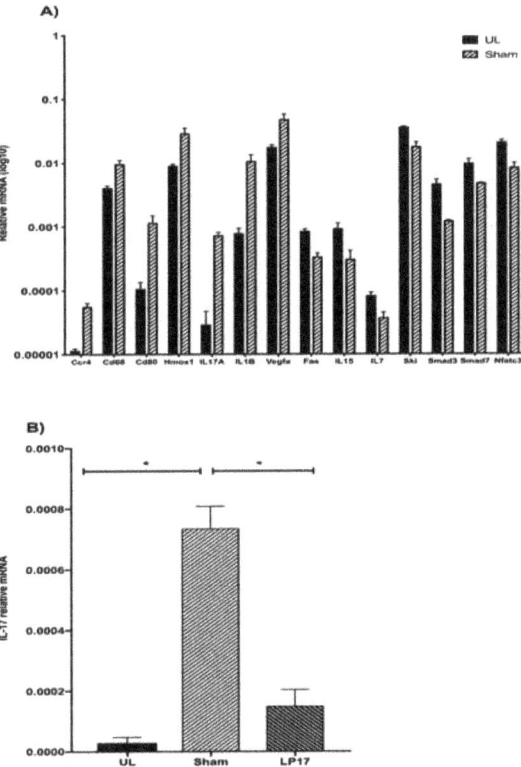

Figure 4. Modulation of immunoregulatory genes by TREM-1. Dissected gingiva from unligated control sites (UL) and ligated sham treated sites (Sham) for 5 days. The mRNA expression of 92 key genes mediating the immune response and four endogenous control genes including *GAPDH, HPRT, GUSB and 18S RNA mRNA* were assessed by qPCR. The gene expression levels were calibrated against the expression of housekeeping genes (detailed list provided in Table S2). The significantly regulated genes are presented (fold-change ≥ 2 and * $p < 0.05$). (**A**). Dissected gingiva from unligated control sites (UL), or ligated sites from PBS sham-treated sites (Sham) or sites treated with 5 μg synthetic TREM-1 inhibitor (LP17) for 5 days. The mRNA expression of IL-17 is presented (fold-change ≥ 2 and * $p < 0.05$). (**B**). Data are means ± SEM (n = 3 mice/group).

Treatment with the LP17 peptide altered the expression of 27 genes by more than two-fold (23 downregulated, 4 upregulated) (Supplement Table S2). Although the expression of proinflammatory cytokines associated with periodontal disease pathogenesis (such as, IL-1β, IL-6, IL-17A, and TNF) was inhibited, statistical significance was reached only for IL-17A, which was downregulated by 4.9-fold (Figure 4B). Taken together, these data indicate that ligature-induced periodontitis is associated with upregulation of a number of proinflammatory genes that seem to be inhibited by LP17, which predominantly targets IL-17A expression, a signature cytokine of Th17 cells that were shown to drive inflammatory bone loss in mice and humans [24].

3.5. Regulation of the RANKL/OPG Axis by TREM-1

The upregulation of IL-17A expression, a cytokine associated with chronic inflammatory tissue destruction and alveolar bone loss [25,26], prompted us to investigate further the involvement of TREM-1 in the molecular regulatory mechanisms of bone resorption, particularly the RANKL/OPG system. RANKL was significantly induced at the sham-treated ligated sites (39-fold), whereas administration of LP17 inhibited this upregulatory effect by 8.9-fold (Figure 5A). The expression of OPG also increased at the sham-treated ligated sites (2.7-fold) but was not significantly affected by administration of LP17 (Figure 5B). As a result, the relative RANKL/OPG ratio, a molecular determinant of bone resorption, was significantly reduced in response to LP17 treatment by five-fold as compared to PBS sham treatment (Figure 5C).

As IL-6 and COX-2 that are produced in high levels during inflammation are considered as key regulators of RANKL expression [4,27,28], we assessed their regulation by TREM-1. Interestingly, the expressions of COX-2 and IL-6 were not significantly affected by LP17 treatment, indicating that the regulation of RANKL in this model may not be dependent on COX-2 (Figure 6A) or IL-6 (Figure 6B).

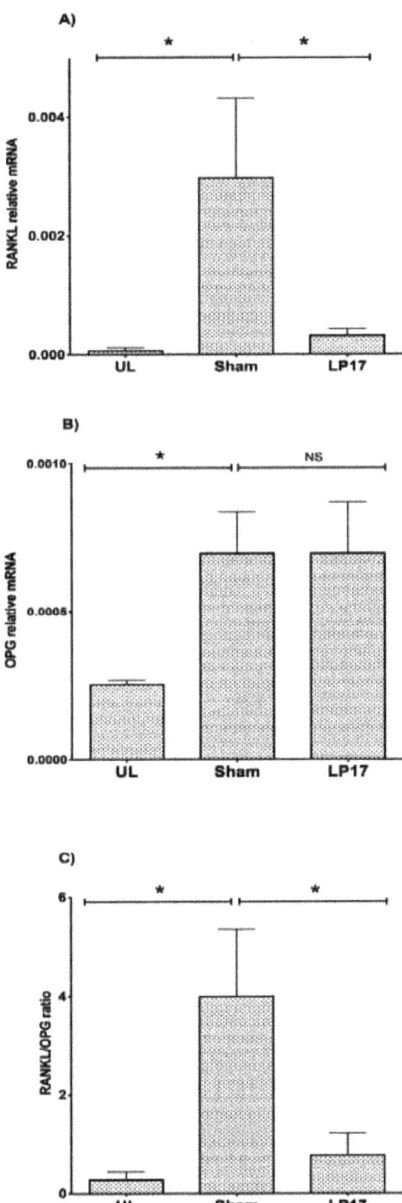

Figure 5. Inhibition of receptor activator of nuclear factor kappa-B-ligand (RANKL)/osteoprotegerin (OPG) ratio by LP17. Gingival tissue samples were dissected at day 5 from mice used in Figure 2 and were processed for gene expression of RANKL (**A**) and OPG (**B**) by qPCR. The relative RANKL/OPG ratio was also calculated (**C**). The expression of the indicated molecules was determined in unligated (UL) control gingiva and in ligated gingival tissues treated with 5 μg synthetic TREM-1 inhibitor (LP17) or PBS sham. The gene expression levels were detected by TaqMan real-time qPCR and calibrated against the expression of the housekeeping gene *β-actin*. Results are means ± SEM (n = 4 mice/group). * $p < 0.05$ and ** $p < 0.01$ between the indicated groups. NS: Not significant, $p > 0.05$.

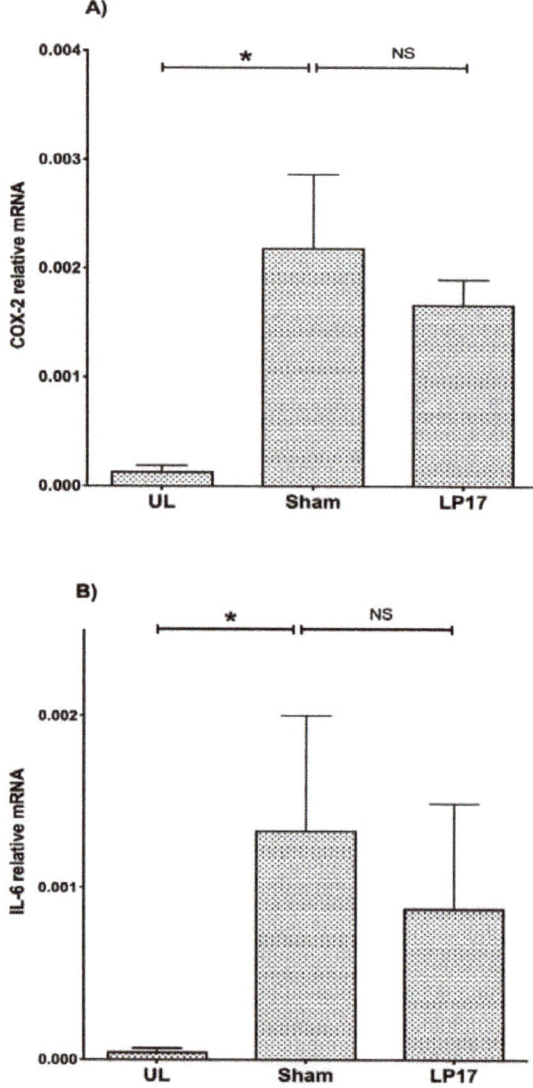

Figure 6. LP17 does not affect COX-2 and IL-6 levels. Gingival tissue samples were dissected at day 5 from mice used in Figure 2 and were processed for gene expression of COX-2 (**A**) and IL-6 (**B**) by qPCR. The expression of the indicated molecules was determined in unligated (UL) control gingiva and in ligated gingival tissues treated with 5 µg synthetic TREM-1 inhibitor (LP17) or PBS sham. The gene expression levels were detected by TaqMan real-time qPCR and calibrated against the expression of the housekeeping gene β-actin. Results are means ± SEM (n = 4 mice/group). NS: Not significant, $p > 0.05$.

4. Discussion

Our present study shows for the first time that TREM-1 regulates alveolar bone loss in experimental periodontitis and paves the way for a novel approach to treat human periodontitis. In line with earlier observations in humans demonstrating upregulated TREM-1 gingival expression in periodontitis patients, as compared to healthy controls [19], our study showed progressively increased induction of TREM-1 gingival expression during the course of experimental periodontitis in response to biofilm accumulation. TREM-1 propagates proinflammatory cytokine expression, representatively demonstrated by IL-1β in the present study. These findings are in accordance with our previous studies showing a positive correlation between subgingival biofilms and TREM-1 levels in gingival tissue or gingival crevicular fluid of individuals with periodontitis [16,19]. Although the cellular distribution of TREM-1 in gingival tissue was not investigated in the present experimental setting, monocytes/resident macrophages and polymorphonuclear neutrophilic leukocytes (PMNs) are known to be a major source of TREM-1 in inflammation [9,29–31]. In this respect, our earlier work presented that multispecies oral biofilms [19] or the keystone pathogen *Porphyromonas gingivalis* is able to induce TREM-1 gene expression in monocytes or in PMNs in the tissue culture systems [20,32].

The major novel finding of this in vivo study is that local (gingival) injection of a TREM-1 blocking peptide, namely LP17, substantially reduced the RANKL/OPG osteoclastogenic ratio and alveolar bone loss, thus providing preclinical support for a new therapeutic target for periodontitis. Clinical studies have demonstrated that the RANKL/OPG ratio as well as IL-17 gingival tissue expression are upregulated in human periodontitis [33–36]. Intriguingly, LP17 selectively downregulated IL-17 expression among all studied immune response markers. Given that IL-17 regulates the expression of RANKL [37], it is possible that the capacity of LP17 to downregulate the RANKL/OPG ratio may be mediated through its ability to inhibit IL-17. Similarly, inhibition of IL-17 by its antagonist Del-1 has been shown to efficiently block osteoclastogenesis and subsequent periodontitis [38,39]. Thus, our study lends further support to the concept that IL-17 is a key driver of periodontal bone loss, although this is the first time that TREM-1 signaling is linked to IL-17 in the context of periodontitis.

Our present data are also consistent with a recent in vitro study, demonstrating that the LR12 TREM-1 inhibitor LR12 could prevent monocytic activation by *P. gingivalis* LPS [40], as well as our earlier in vitro findings demonstrating that LP17 can reduce cytokine release by monocytes in response to *P. gingivalis* whole bacteria [20,21]. Moreover, an earlier study in a psoriasis model showed that TREM-1 blockade in vitro and ex vivo significantly reduced the number of Th17 cells and decreased the secretion of IL-17, suggesting that TREM-1 positively regulates Th17 responses [41]. The COX-2 pathway and IL-6 are also important regulators of the RANKL/OPG ratio [27]. However, it is unlikely that TREM-1 regulates the RANKL/OPG ratio via COX-2 or IL-6 since LP17 failed to affect the expression of either gene. Thus, it is concluded that the alveolar bone resorptive effects of TREM-1 are, at least in part, mediated through activation of the IL-17-RANKL axis.

Although the impact of TREM-1 signaling on microbial control has been controversial in several bacterial challenge models [13], in the experimental periodontitis model, LP17 did not show a significant effect on oral bacterial load. This finding suggests that TREM-1 inhibition protects against periodontitis predominantly through host-modulation effects and is in line with earlier work indicating that LP17 did not alter the in vitro levels of *P. gingivalis* [20,32,42].

Moreover, TREM-1-deficient mice used in colitis and other experimental models of infection-driven inflammatory diseases exhibited no alterations in microbial clearance efficiency [13]. On the other hand, studies on lung infection models (e.g., *Pseudomonas aeruginosa*-induced pneumonia) indicated that administration of LP17 peptide reduced the bacterial load at an early stage of infection while increasing it at later stages; these effects, however, were attributed to indirect antimicrobial effects of TREM-1 related to early enhancement of neutrophil influx and consequent increase in phagocytic activity [43]. These observations are in line with the main function of TREM-1 as an inflammation fine-tuner [44], rather than a direct eliminator of infection, as is the case, for instance, for TNF-alpha. Yet, the use of anti-TNF antibody may be complicated because of the increased risk for reactivation of latent infection [45].

5. Conclusions

The present study conclusively demonstrated the involvement of TREM-1 in alveolar bone resorption during the course of experimental periodontitis in mice. Mechanistically, TREM-1 reduced the RANKL/OPG osteoclastogenic ratio, presumably via the inhibition of IL-17. Importantly, our findings also reveal a previously unidentified TREM-1-driven axis for inflammatory bone loss that could be targeted via small-molecule antagonists for therapeutic intervention in human periodontitis.

Supplementary Materials: The following are available online at http://www.mdpi.com/2077-0383/8/10/1579/s1, Table S1: Immune gene expression profile in ligated gingiva vs healthy gingiva, Table S2: immune regulatory genes in mouse gingiva by LP17.

Author Contributions: Conceptualization, N.B. and G.H.; Methodology, N.B., T.A,. G.N.B., and N.B.; Validation, N.B., G.N.B. and G.H.; Formal Analysis, T.A., N.B.; Resources, N.B., G.N.B., G.H.; Writing—Original Draft Preparation, N.B.; Writing—Review & Editing, G.H., G.N.B.; Visualization, T.A.; Supervision, G.H.; Funding Acquisition, N.B., G.N.B. and G.H.

Funding: This research was funded by grants from the National Institutes of Health (DE015254, DE024716, DE024153, and DE026152 to G.H.), the Swedish Research Council funds (2017-01198 to N.B.), and the APC by strategic funds from Karolinska Institutet (G.N.B.).

Conflicts of Interest: The authors declare no conflicts of interest.

References

1. Lamont, R.J.; Hajishengallis, G. Polymicrobial synergy and dysbiosis in inflammatory disease. *Trends Mol. Med.* **2015**, *21*, 172–183. [CrossRef] [PubMed]
2. Hajishengallis, G.; Korostoff, J.M. Revisiting the Page & Schroeder model: The good, the bad and the unknowns in the periodontal host response 40 years later. *Periodontol. 2000* **2017**, *75*, 116–151. [PubMed]
3. Garlet, G.P. Destructive and Protective Roles of Cytokines in Periodontitis: A Re-appraisal from Host Defense and Tissue Destruction Viewpoints. *J. Dent. Res.* **2010**, *89*, 1349–1363. [CrossRef] [PubMed]
4. Lerner, U. Inflammation-induced bone remodeling in periodontal disease and the influence of post-menopausal osteoporosis. *J. Dent. Res.* **2006**, *85*, 596–607. [CrossRef] [PubMed]
5. Belibasakis, G.N.; Bostanci, N. The RANKL-OPG system in clinical periodontology. *J. Clin. Periodontol.* **2012**, *39*, 239–248. [CrossRef] [PubMed]
6. Belibasakis, G.N.; Meier, A.; Guggenheim, B.; Bostanci, N. The RANKL-OPG system is differentially regulated by supragingival and subgingival biofilm supernatants. *Cytokine* **2011**, *55*, 98–103. [CrossRef]
7. Gibot, S.; Cravoisy, A. Soluble Form of the Triggering Receptor Expressed on Myeloid Cells-1 as a Marker of Microbial Infection. *Clin. Med. Res.* **2004**, *2*, 181–187. [CrossRef]
8. Colonna, M.; Facchetti, F. TREM-1 (Triggering Receptor Expressed on Myeloid Cells): A New Player in Acute Inflammatory Responses. *J. Infect. Dis.* **2003**, *187*, S397–S401. [CrossRef]
9. Schenk, M.; Bouchon, A.; Seibold, F.; Mueller, C. TREM-1–expressing intestinal macrophages crucially amplify chronic inflammation in experimental colitis and inflammatory bowel diseases. *J. Clin. Investig.* **2007**, *117*, 3097–3106. [CrossRef]
10. Gibot, S.; Kolopp-Sarda, M.-N.; Bene, M.-C.; Bollaert, P.-E.; Lozniewski, A.; Mory, F.; Lévy, B.; Faure, G.C. A Soluble Form of the Triggering Receptor Expressed on Myeloid Cells-1 Modulates the Inflammatory Response in Murine Sepsis. *J. Exp. Med.* **2004**, *200*, 1419–1426. [CrossRef]
11. Bouchon, A.; Facchetti, F.; Weigand, M.A.; Colonna, M. TREM-1 amplifies inflammation and is a crucial mediator of septic shock. *Nature* **2001**, *410*, 1103–1107. [CrossRef] [PubMed]
12. Boechat, N.; Bouchonnet, F.; Bonay, M.; Grodet, A.; Pelicic, V.; Gicquel, B.; Hance, A.J. Culture at High Density Improves the Ability of Human Macrophages to Control Mycobacterial Growth. *J. Immunol.* **2001**, *166*, 6203–6211. [CrossRef] [PubMed]
13. Weber, B.; Schuster, S.; Zysset, D.; Rihs, S.; Dickgreber, N.; Schurch, C.; Riether, C.; Siegrist, M.; Schneider, C.; Pawelski, H.; et al. TREM-1 Deficiency Can Attenuate Disease Severity without Affecting Pathogen Clearance. *PLoS Pathog.* **2014**, *10*, e1003900. [CrossRef] [PubMed]

14. Bostanci, N.; Öztürk, V.Ö.; Emingil, G.; Belibasakis, G.N. Elevated oral and systemic levels of soluble triggering receptor expressed on myeloid cells-1 (sTREM-1) in periodontitis. *J. Dent. Res.* **2013**, *92*, 161–165. [CrossRef] [PubMed]
15. Nylund, K.M.; Ruokonen, H.; Sorsa, T.; Heikkinen, A.M.; Meurman, J.H.; Ortiz, F.; Tervahartiala, T.; Furuholm, J.; Bostanci, N. Association of the Salivary Triggering Receptor Expressed on Myeloid Cells/its Ligand Peptidoglycan Recognition Protein 1 Axis with Oral Inflammation in Kidney Disease. *J. Periodontol.* **2018**, *89*, 117–129. [CrossRef]
16. Belibasakis, G.N.; Öztürk, V.; Emingil, G.; Bostanci, N. Soluble Triggering Receptor Expressed on Myeloid Cells 1 (sTREM-1) in Gingival Crevicular Fluid: Association with Clinical and Microbiologic Parameters. *J. Periodontol.* **2014**, *85*, 204–210. [CrossRef]
17. Bisson, C.; Massin, F.; Lefevre, P.A.; Thilly, N.; Miller, N.; Gibot, S. Increased gingival crevicular fluid levels of soluble triggering receptor expressed on myeloid cells (sTREM) -1 in severe periodontitis. *J. Clin. Periodontol.* **2012**, *39*, 1141–1148. [CrossRef]
18. Öztürk, V.Ö.; Belibasakis, G.N.; Emingil, G.; Bostanci, N. Impact of aging on TREM-1 responses in the periodontium: A cross-sectional study in an elderly population. *BMC Infect. Dis.* **2016**, *16*, 429.
19. Willi, M.; Belibasakis, G.N.; Bostanci, N. Expression and regulation of triggering receptor expressed on myeloid cells 1 in periodontal diseases. *Clin. Exp. Immunol.* **2014**, *178*, 190–200. [CrossRef]
20. Bostanci, N.; Thurnheer, T.; Belibasakis, G.N. Involvement of the TREM-1/DAP12 pathway in the innate immune responses to Porphyromonas gingivalis. *Mol. Immunol.* **2011**, *49*, 387–394. [CrossRef]
21. Bostanci, N.; Belibasakis, G.N. Doxycycline inhibits TREM-1 induction by Porphyromonas gingivalis. *FEMS Immunol. Med. Microbiol.* **2012**, *66*, 37–44. [CrossRef] [PubMed]
22. Abe, T.; Hajishengallis, G. Optimization of the ligature-induced periodontitis model in mice. *J. Immunol. Methods* **2013**, *394*, 49–54. [CrossRef] [PubMed]
23. Pelham, C.J.; Pandya, A.N.; Agrawal, D.K. Triggering receptor expressed on myeloid cells receptor family modulators: A patent review. *Expert Opin. Ther. Patents* **2014**, *24*, 1383–1395. [CrossRef] [PubMed]
24. Dutzan, N.; Kajikawa, T.; Abusleme, L.; Greenwell-Wild, T.; Zuazo, C.E.; Ikeuchi, T.; Brenchley, L.; Abe, T.; Hurabielle, C.; Martin, D.; et al. A dysbiotic microbiome triggers TH17 cells to mediate oral mucosal immunopathology in mice and humans. *Sci. Transl. Med.* **2018**, *10*, 0797. [CrossRef] [PubMed]
25. Gaffen, S.; Hajishengallis, G. A new inflammatory cytokine on the block: Re-thinking periodontal disease and the Th1/Th2 paradigm in the context of Th17 cells and IL-17. *J. Dent. Res.* **2008**, *87*, 817–828. [CrossRef] [PubMed]
26. Zenobia, C.; Hajishengallis, G. Basic biology and role of interleukin-17 in immunity and inflammation. *Periodontol. 2000* **2015**, *69*, 142–159. [CrossRef]
27. Belibasakis, G.N.; Guggenheim, B. Induction of prostaglandin E 2 and interleukin-6 in gingival fibroblasts by oral biofilms. *FEMS Immunol. Med. Microbiol.* **2011**, *63*, 381–386. [CrossRef] [PubMed]
28. Reddi, D.; Bostanci, N.; Hashim, A.; Aduse-Opoku, J.; Curtis, M.A.; Hughes, F.J.; Belibasakis, G.N. Porphyromonas gingivalis regulates the RANKL-OPG system in bone marrow stromal cells. *Microbes Infect.* **2008**, *10*, 1459–1468. [CrossRef]
29. Arts, R.J.; Joosten, L.A.; Dinarello, C.A.; Kullberg, B.J.; Van Der Meer, J.W.; Netea, M.G. TREM-1 interaction with the LPS/TLR4 receptor complex. *Eur. Cytokine Netw.* **2011**, *22*, 11–14. [CrossRef]
30. Alflen, A.; Stadler, N.; Lopez, P.A.; Teschner, D.; Theobald, M.; Heß, G.; Radsak, M.P. Idelalisib impairs TREM-1 mediated neutrophil inflammatory responses. *Sci. Rep.* **2018**, *8*, 5558. [CrossRef]
31. Fortin, C.F.; Lesur, O.; Fulop, T., Jr. Effects of TREM-1 activation in human neutrophils: Activation of signaling pathways, recruitment into lipid rafts and association with TLR4. *Int. Immunol.* **2007**, *19*, 41–50. [CrossRef] [PubMed]
32. Bostanci, N.; Thurnheer, T.; Aduse-Opoku, J.; Curtis, M.A.; Zinkernagel, A.S.; Belibasakis, G.N. Porphyromonas gingivalis Regulates TREM-1 in Human Polymorphonuclear Neutrophils via Its Gingipains. *PLoS ONE* **2013**, *8*, e75784. [CrossRef] [PubMed]
33. Takahashi, K.; Azuma, T.; Motohira, H.; Kinane, D.F.; Kitetsu, S. The potential role of interleukin-17 in the immunopathology of periodontal disease. *J. Clin. Periodontol.* **2005**, *32*, 369–374. [CrossRef] [PubMed]
34. Bostanci, N.; Ilgenli, T.; Emingil, G.; Afacan, B.; Han, B.; Töz, H.; Berdeli, A.; Atilla, G.; McKay, I.J.; Hughes, F.J.; et al. Differential expression of receptor activator of nuclear factor-kappaB ligand and osteoprotegerin mRNA in periodontal diseases. *J. Periodontal Res.* **2007**, *42*, 287–293. [CrossRef] [PubMed]

35. Dutzan, N.; Konkel, J.E.; Greenwell-Wild, T.; Moutsopoulos, N.M. Characterization of the human immune cell network at the gingival barrier. *Mucosal Immunol.* **2016**, *9*, 1163–1172. [CrossRef]
36. Moutsopoulos, N.M.; Konkel, J.; Sarmadi, M.; Eskan, M.A.; Wild, T.; Dutzan, N.; Abusleme, L.; Zenobia, C.; Hosur, K.B.; Abe, T.; et al. Defective neutrophil recruitment in leukocyte adhesion deficiency type I disease causes local IL-17-driven inflammatory bone loss. *Sci. Transl. Med.* **2014**, *6*, 229ra40. [CrossRef]
37. Koenders, M.I.; Lubberts, E.; Oppers-Walgreen, B.; Bersselaar, L.V.D.; Helsen, M.M.; Di Padova, F.E.; Boots, A.M.; Gram, H.; Joosten, L.A.; Berg, W.B. Blocking of Interleukin-17 during Reactivation of Experimental Arthritis Prevents Joint Inflammation and Bone Erosion by Decreasing RANKL and Interleukin-1. *Am. J. Pathol.* **2005**, *167*, 141–149. [CrossRef]
38. Shin, J.; Maekawa, T.; Abe, T.; Hajishengallis, E.; Hosur, K.; Pyaram, K.; Mitroulis, I.; Chavakis, T.; Hajishengallis, G. DEL-1 restrains osteoclastogenesis and inhibits inflammatory bone loss in nonhuman primates. *Sci. Transl. Med.* **2015**, *7*, 307ra155. [CrossRef]
39. Eskan, M.A.; Jotwani, R.; Abe, T.; Chmelar, J.; Lim, J.-H.; Liang, S.; Ciero, P.A.; Krauss, J.L.; Li, F.; Rauner, M.; et al. The leukocyte integrin antagonist Del-1 inhibits IL-17-mediated inflammatory bone loss. *Nat. Immunol.* **2012**, *13*, 465–473. [CrossRef]
40. Dubar, M.; Carrasco, K.; Gibot, S.; Bisson, C. Effects of Porphyromonas gingivalis LPS and LR12 peptide on TREM-1 expression by monocytes. *J. Clin. Periodontol.* **2018**, *45*, 799–805. [CrossRef]
41. Hyder, L.A.; Gonzalez, J.; Harden, J.L.; Johnson-Huang, L.M.; Zaba, L.C.; Pierson, K.C.; Eungdamrong, N.J.; Lentini, T.; Gulati, N.; Fuentes-Duculan, J.; et al. TREM-1 as a potential therapeutic target in psoriasis. *J. Investig. Dermatol.* **2013**, *133*, 1742–1751. [CrossRef]
42. Hajishengallis, G.; Liang, S.; Payne, M.A.; Hashim, A.; Jotwani, R.; Eskan, M.A.; McIntosh, M.L.; Alsam, A.; Kirkwood, K.L.; Lambris, J.D.; et al. Low-abundance biofilm species orchestrates inflammatory periodontal disease through the commensal microbiota and complement. *Cell Host Microbe* **2011**, *10*, 497–506. [CrossRef] [PubMed]
43. Klesney-Tait, J.; Keck, K.; Li, X.; Gilfillan, S.; Otero, K.; Baruah, S.; Meyerholz, D.K.; Varga, S.M.; Knudson, C.J.; Moninger, T.O.; et al. Transepithelial migration of neutrophils into the lung requires TREM-1. *J. Clin. Investig.* **2013**, *123*, 138–149. [CrossRef] [PubMed]
44. Silbereisen, A.; Hallak, A.; Nascimento, G.; Sorsa, T.; Belibasakis, G.; Lopez, R.; Bostanci, N. Regulation of PGLYRP1 and TREM-1 during Progression and Resolution of Gingival Inflammation. *JDR Clin. Transl. Res.* **2019**, *4*, 352–359. [CrossRef]
45. Keane, J.; Gershon, S.; Wise, R.P.; Mirabile-Levens, E.; Kasznica, J.; Schwieterman, W.D.; Siegel, J.N.; Braun, M.M. Tuberculosis associated with infliximab, a tumor necrosis factor alpha-neutralizing agent. *N. Engl. J. Med.* **2001**, *345*, 1098–1104. [CrossRef] [PubMed]

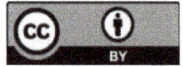

© 2019 by the authors. Licensee MDPI, Basel, Switzerland. This article is an open access article distributed under the terms and conditions of the Creative Commons Attribution (CC BY) license (http://creativecommons.org/licenses/by/4.0/).

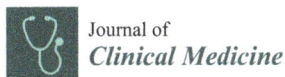

Article

Saliva and Serum Immune Responses in Apical Periodontitis

Milla Pietiäinen [1,*], John M. Liljestrand [1,*], Ramin Akhi [2,3,4,*], Kåre Buhlin [1,5], Anders Johansson [6], Susanna Paju [1], Aino Salminen [1], Päivi Mäntylä [7,8], Juha Sinisalo [9], Leo Tjäderhane [1], Sohvi Hörkkö [2,3,4] and Pirkko J. Pussinen [1]

[1] Oral and Maxillofacial Diseases, University of Helsinki and Helsinki University Hospital, FI-00014 Helsinki, Finland; kare.buhlin@ki.se (K.B.); susanna.paju@helsinki.fi (S.P.); aino.m.salminen@helsinki.fi (A.S.); leo.tjaderhane@helsinki.fi (L.T.); pirkko.pussinen@helsinki.fi (P.J.P.)
[2] Medical Microbiology and Immunology, Research Unit of Biomedicine, University of Oulu, FI-90014 Oulu, Finland; sohvi.horkko@nordlab.fi
[3] Medical Research Center, Oulu University Hospital and University of Oulu, FI-90014 Oulu, Finland
[4] Nordlab, Oulu University Hospital, FI-90220 Oulu, Finland
[5] Division of Periodontology, Department of Dental Medicine, Karolinska Institutet, S-141 04 Huddinge, Sweden
[6] Department of Odontology, Molecular Periodontology Research, Umeå University, S-901 87 Umeå, Sweden; anders.p.johansson@umu.se
[7] Institute of Dentistry, University of Eastern Finland, FI-70211 Kuopio, Finland; paivi.mantyla@uef.fi
[8] Kuopio University Hospital, Oral and Maxillofacial Diseases, FI-70029 Kuopio, Finland
[9] HUCH Heart and Lung Center, Helsinki University Hospital, FI-00029 Helsinki, Finland; juha.sinisalo@hus.fi
* Correspondence: milla.pietiainen@helsinki.fi (M.P.); john.liljestrand@helsinki.fi (J.M.L.); ramin.akhi@oulu.fi (R.A.)

Received: 10 June 2019; Accepted: 17 June 2019; Published: 21 June 2019

Abstract: Apical periodontitis is an inflammatory reaction at the apex of an infected tooth. Its microbiota resembles that of marginal periodontitis and may induce local and systemic antibodies binding to bacteria- and host-derived epitopes. Our aim was to investigate the features of the adaptive immune response in apical periodontitis. The present Parogene cohort ($n = 453$) comprises patients with cardiac symptoms. Clinical and radiographic oral examination was performed to diagnose apical and marginal periodontitis. A three-category endodontic lesion score was designed. Antibodies binding to the bacteria- and host-derived epitopes were determined from saliva and serum, and bacterial compositions were examined from saliva and subgingival samples. The significant ORs (95% CI) for the highest endodontic scores were observed for saliva IgA and IgG to bacterial antigens (2.90 (1.01–8.33) and 4.91 (2.48–9.71)/log10 unit), saliva cross-reacting IgG (2.10 (1.48–2.97)), serum IgG to bacterial antigens (4.66 (1.22–10.1)), and Gram-negative subgingival species (1.98 (1.16–3.37)). In a subgroup without marginal periodontitis, only saliva IgG against bacterial antigens associated with untreated apical periodontitis (4.77 (1.05–21.7)). Apical periodontitis associates with versatile adaptive immune responses against both bacterial- and host-derived epitopes independently of marginal periodontitis. Saliva immunoglobulins could be useful biomarkers of oral infections including apical periodontitis—a putative risk factor for systemic diseases.

Keywords: apical periodontitis; adaptive immunity; saliva; serum; antibody

1. Introduction

Apical periodontitis (AP) is an inflammatory disease that affects the tissues surrounding the apex of the tooth. It is triggered by oral pathogens infecting root canal. Both acute (abscess) and chronic inflammatory reaction (periapical granuloma and radicular cyst) can develop depending on the intensity of the bacterial infection and the host immune responses. Primary apical periodontitis usually develops when the bacteria in a caries lesion enter through enamel and dentin and cause microbial colonization of the pulp and eventually necrosis of the pulp tissue. Secondary apical periodontitis arises from a persistent infection of previously treated root canals or leakage of the filling in a root canal-treated tooth. Apical periodontitis is diagnosed from radiographs as an evident radiolucent area (referred to as endodontic lesion) at the tip of the root. Even slight radiographically evident widening of the periapical space is associated with an infection in the tooth [1]. AP is treated with root canal treatment where infection is eliminated chemomechanically and the root canal is filled.

Apical periodontitis is a highly common and underdiagnosed disease. It is estimated that approximately 10% of all teeth are endodontically treated, 5% have periapical radiolucencies [2], and the prevalence of apical periodontitis varies between 24 and 86% in different populations [3]. Up to 78% of endodontically treated teeth have root canal fillings with poor quality and ~36% of the root canal-treated teeth present apical periodontitis [2], suggesting that recurrent or persistent endodontic infections are common. Apical periodontitis is usually symptomless, and it can be diagnosed only by radiography.

Endodontic infections are polymicrobial and the structure of the intracanal biofilm may evolve toward obligate aerobes and Gram-negative anaerobes as the infection progresses. More than 400 different microbial taxa have been identified in endodontic samples from teeth with different forms of apical periodontitis [4]. Several studies have also shown that distinct bacterial communities are found in primary and secondary AP [5–8]. Despite the high interindividual variability in endodontic microbial community composition, the most often encountered phyla in the intracanal samples include Firmicutes, Actinobacteria, Bacteroidetes, Proteobacteria, and Fusobacteria. Genera such as Prevotella, Fusobacterium, Parvimonas, Lactobacillus, Streptococcus, and Porphyromonas are highly prevalent in intracanal samples [9]. Several members of these genera are also considered etiological pathogens for marginal periodontitis and the microbial profiles of these two conditions resemble each other [10].

Microbial antigens stimulate innate immune responses in periapical tissue aiming to restrict the infection. The expression of proinflammatory cytokines, prostaglandins, and proteolytic enzymes are markedly increased in the areas of tissue destruction [11]. As one antimicrobial strategy, apical periodontitis is also associated with oxidative stress [12]. Some studies suggest a modest contribution of endodontic infections to the plasmatic inflammatory markers [13,14], while a recent study found a significant association between endodontic lesions and systemic inflammatory burden in young adults [15].

Additionally, adaptive immune responses are activated to prevent the microbial invasion into the tissues surrounding teeth or into circulation. High concentrations of local immunoglobulins IgG and IgA and lesser amounts of IgM and secretory IgA are present in the inflamed tissues [16–19]. The levels of systemic immunoglobulins, including total IgA, IgG, and IgM, are increased in patients with AP [13]. We recently showed that subgingival *Porphyromonas endodontalis* levels and serum IgG against it were associated with a higher endodontic lesion score [20]. Several oral pathogens are also known to be able to induce cross-reactive antibodies, which may influence inflammatory responses. The cross-reactive antibodies are part of an immunological process called molecular mimicry, in which bacterial antigens sufficiently resembling human proteins are able to induce the production of antibodies reacting with human epitopes. The most studied epitopes include those present in the heat shock proteins (HSPs) and in oxidized low-density lipoproteins (oxLDL) [21].

The association of marginal periodontitis with several systemic conditions such as cardiovascular diseases (CVDs) is well established [22]. Due to similarities in the inflammatory and microbial profiles between marginal periodontitis and AP, it is also suggested that there could be a link between AP and CVDs [23,24]. Even though the possible association of apical periodontitis with systemic diseases has been of high interest, the adaptive immune response against the disease has not been investigated in detail. In this study we aimed to investigate serum and saliva antibodies against several oral pathogens associated with apical periodontitis and the role of cross-reactive antibodies in the disease.

2. Experimental Section

2.1. Population

The Corogene is a prospective cohort of Finnish patients who had an indication to coronary angiography between June 2006 and March 2008 at the Helsinki University Hospital [25]. The present study comprises the Parogene, which is a substudy of 508 patients with clinical and radiographic oral health examinations. The details of the examinations have been described elsewhere [26]. The information of smoking habits was collected with a questionnaire before the oral examination. The presence of diabetes (type I and II) was obtained from medical records. All subjects signed an informed consent and the study was approved by the Helsinki University Hospital ethics committee (approval reference number 106/2007). Patients with antibody measurements from serum and saliva samples were included ($n = 453$, 89.2% of the whole cohort). The number of dentate patients and subgingival samples was 426 (n of edentulous 27, 6.0%).

2.2. Oral Diagnosis

Endodontic lesions were diagnosed from the radiographs as described in detail earlier [20]. The recorded findings included root canal fillings, widened periapical space indicating irreversible pulpitis or precursors for endodontic lesions [1], and apical periodontitis seen as periradicular destruction in the tip of the root. An endodontic lesion score was defined to describe the severity of apical periodontitis [20]. Score I included patients without endodontic lesions ($n = 162$, 38.2%); score II, patients with ≥1 widened periapical space and/or 1 tooth with apical periodontitis ($n = 194$, 45.2%); and score III, patients with ≥2 teeth with apical periodontitis ($n = 68$, 16.0%). In addition, another subgrouping—the endodontic treatment score—was designed according to treated/untreated apical periodontitis: I, no endodontic lesions ($n = 352$, 77.7%); II, teeth with apical periodontitis, all with root canal fillings ($n = 51$, 11.3%); and III, apical periodontitis in tooth/teeth without root canal fillings ($n = 50$, 11.0%). Number of teeth and implants, presence of carious teeth, and inadequate root canal fillings were also recorded from the radiographs.

Diagnosis for marginal periodontitis was based on alveolar bone loss (ABL) detected in the radiographs and bleeding on probing (BOP) registered in the clinical examination from four sites of each tooth. Patient was considered periodontally healthy, when no ABL and <25% BOP was present; with gingivitis, when no ABL but ≥25% BOP; and with periodontitis, when ABL was present [27].

2.3. Bacterial Analyses

Subgingival plaque samples were collected from the deepest pathological periodontal pocket (≥ 4 mm) in each dentate quadrant as described earlier [28]. The microbiome analysis including 79 taxa was performed by using the checkerboard DNA-DNA hybridization assay [29] and the data was analyzed as described in our earlier article [28]. In the present work, we summed up the results of Gram-positive taxa ($n = 45$) and Gram-negative taxa ($n = 34$), which are presented in Supplementary Table S1.

Saliva samples were collected after stimulation by chewing for 5 min, and a minimum of 2 mL of saliva was collected by expectoration. The methods for sample processing and quantitative real-time PCR have been described in detail earlier [30]. Saliva concentration of four bacterial species associated with periodontitis was analyzed: *Aggregatibacter actinomycetemcomitans*, *Porphyromonas gingivalis*, *Tannerella forsythia*, and *Prevotella intermedia*.

2.4. Antibody Determinations

Serum IgA- and IgG-class antibody levels against seven bacterial species—*A. actinomycetemcomitans, P. gingivalis, T. forsythia, P. intermedia, Campylobacter rectus, Fusobacterium nucleatum,* and *P. endodontalis*—were determined with ELISA as described earlier [31]. The antigens were composed of formalin-killed whole cells and two dilutions in duplicate were measured [32]. After all antibody levels were determined, the absorbances were normalized according to the reference applied on each plate and the results were expressed as continuous ELISA-units (EU). The list of the antigens, sample dilutions, and coefficients of interassay variations are presented earlier [31].

Saliva IgA- and IgG-class antibody levels against five species—*A. actinomycetemcomitans, P. gingivalis, T. forsythia, P. intermedia,* and *P. endodontalis*—were determined from saliva supernatants obtained after centrifugation at 9300× *g* for 3 min. The target antigens used in the assays were either heat-killed whole bacterial cells or oxidized LDL epitope malondialdehyde acetaldehyde modification (MAA-LDL), copper-oxidized LDL (CuOx-LDL) [33], recombinant *P. gingivalis* virulence factor gingipain (Rgp44) [34], and 60-kDa *A. actinomycetemcomitans* heat shock protein (Aa-HSP60) [35]. Levels of salivary IgA and IgG antibodies to oxidized LDL and bacterial epitopes were determined by chemiluminescence immunoassay as previously described in detail [36,37]. The saliva samples were diluted accordingly: 1:250 for total IgA and IgG, 1:50 for IgA to oxidized antigens, 1:20 for Aa-HSP60, and 1:10 for bacterial antigens. For IgG measurements, saliva samples were diluted 1:10 for all antigens. Each saliva sample was measured as triplicates. Immunoassay results were presented as relative light units (RLU) per 100 milliseconds (ms).

2.5. Calculations of Cross-Reactive Antibodies and Antibodies Binding to Bacterial Antigens

In addition to the mean levels of antibodies against each specific antigen, the combined antibody levels of saliva and serum IgA and IgG were calculated. The bacterial antigens included *A. actinomycetemcomitans, P. gingivalis, P. intermedia, P. endodontalis,* and *T. forsythia* (referred as IgA/IgG against bacteria). The epitopes recognized in *P. gingivalis* and *A. actinomycetemcomitans* giving rise to cross-reactive antibodies with MAA-LDL included Rgp-44 and Aa-HSP60 (referred as cross-reacting IgA/IgG).

2.6. Statistical Methods

The characteristics are presented as mean values with standard deviations (SD) or 95% confidence intervals. For clarity, standard error is displayed in the figures as error bars. In the supplementary tables, the bacterial levels are presented as medians and interquartile ranges (IQR). Before statistical comparisons, the antibody and bacterial levels were transformed with 10-base logarithm. The significance of the differences was tested by using *t*-test, ANOVA, Chi-square, or Mann–Whitney, when appropriate. The weighted linear terms were examined with ANOVA and Jonckheere–Terpstra test for normally distributed and skewed data, respectively. The associations were analyzed by using linear and logistic regression models adjusted for age, sex, marginal periodontitis (healthy, gingivitis, and periodontitis), number of teeth, and smoking (never/ever). When the dependent variable was composed of several subgroups, multinomial regression was used. When the associations were examined in the subgroup of patients without marginal periodontitis, the confounders were limited to age, sex, and smoking (never/ever).

3. Results

Characteristics of the dentate population are presented in Table 1. The mean (SD) age was 62.9 (9.1) years and 67% were males. The mean number of teeth was 21.4 (7.5), and caries and apical periodontitis were common findings, in 47.4% and 23.8% of the population, respectively. Also, marginal periodontitis ranging from mild to severe was present in most patients (75.5%).

Table 1. Characteristics of the population.

Character	Mean (SD)
Age (years)	62.9 (9.1)
BMI (kg/m^2)	27.8 (5.1)
Number of teeth	21.4 (7.5)
	Mean (95% CI)
Number of implants	0.12 (0.05–0.18)
Carious teeth	0.99 (0.84–1.14)
Root canal fillings	2.17 (1.96–2.39)
Inadequate root fillings	1.08 (0.95–1.20)
Widened periapical space	0.80 (0.71–0.89)
Apical periodontitis	0.36 (0.27–0.45)
With root canal fillings	0.16 (0.12–0.21)
Without root canal fillings	0.19 (0.11–0.27)
	N (%)
Gender (males)	284 (67.0)
Smoking (ever)	220 (51.9)
Hypertension	266 (62.9)
Diabetes (type I or II)	92 (21.9)
Dyslipidemia	340 (80.6)
Carious teeth	198 (47.4)
Root canal fillings	304 (71.7)
Widened periapical spaces	224 (53.8)
Apical periodontitis	101 (23.8)
Endodontic lesion score — No endodontic lesions	162 (38.2)
≥1 tooth with widened periapical space or one tooth with apical periodontitis	194 (45.8)
≥2 teeth with apical periodontitis	68 (16.0)
Endodontic treatment score — No endodontic lesions	323 (76.2)
Apical periodontitis in teeth with root canal fillings	51 (12.0)
Apical periodontitis in teeth without root canal fillings	50 (11.8)
Marginal periodontitis — Healthy	42 (9.9)
Gingivitis	61 (14.4)
Periodontitis	320 (75.5)

The endodontic findings registered included root canal fillings, widened periapical space, and apical periodontitis. Mean antibody levels in serum and saliva against specific antigens, as well as the saliva and subgingival bacterial levels according to the endodontic findings are presented in supplementary tables (Supplementary Tables S2 and S3).

Among serum or saliva IgA-class antibody levels only sporadic significant differences were observed between patients with and without endodontic findings, whereas among IgG-class antibodies several significant differences were found. The antigens producing these differences included *A. actinomycetemcomitans, P. gingivalis, P. intermedia, P. endodontalis, C. rectus, F. nucleatum,* and *T. forsythia*, as well as Aa-HSP60, rgp44, MAA-LDL, and CuOx-LDL (Table S2). Among the salivary or subgingival bacterial concentrations, significant differences were mostly found between patients with and without widened periapical spaces (Table S3).

For further analyses, the microbial biomarkers were combined, and the mean levels are presented in Figures 1 and 2. The combinations included antibody level against bacteria, cross-reactive antibodies, salivary bacteria, and subgingival bacteria. Similarly as above, the mean saliva IgG-class antibody levels against bacteria and the cross-reactive antibodies as well as saliva and subgingival bacterial levels were higher in patients with endodontic findings. From the serum antibody levels, the IgG against bacteria were higher only in patients with widened periapical spaces ($p = 0.015$). In these patients, the increase of subgingival bacterial levels was due to both Gram-positive ($p = 0.022$) and Gram-negative ($p = 0.005$) species.

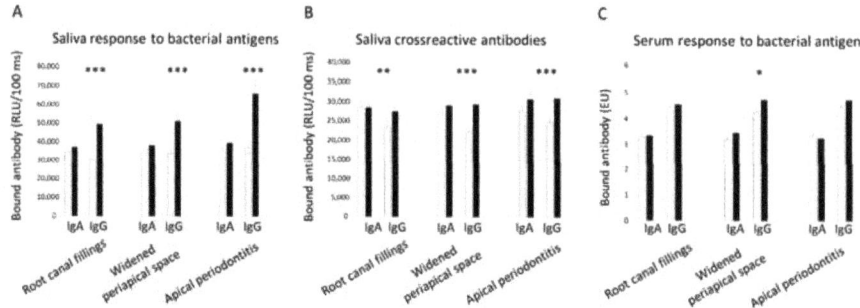

Figure 1. Saliva and serum antibody levels according to endodontic findings. The patients were divided into groups according to the presence of root canal fillings, widened periapical spaces, and apical periodontitis. Saliva (A, B) and serum (C) IgA- and IgG-class antibodies were determined. The bacterial antigens included *A. actinomycetemcomitans*, *P. gingivalis*, *P. intermedia*, *P. endodontalis*, and *T. forsythia*. The antigens giving rise to cross-reactive antibodies included MAA-LDL, Rgp-44, and Aa-HSP60. White columns depict the absence of the endodontic finding and black columns depict the presence of the endodontic finding. Means and standard errors are shown. The asterisks depict statistical significance between the groups defined by the *t*-test after logarithmic transformation: * $p < 0.05$, ** $p < 0.01$. *** $p < 0.001$.

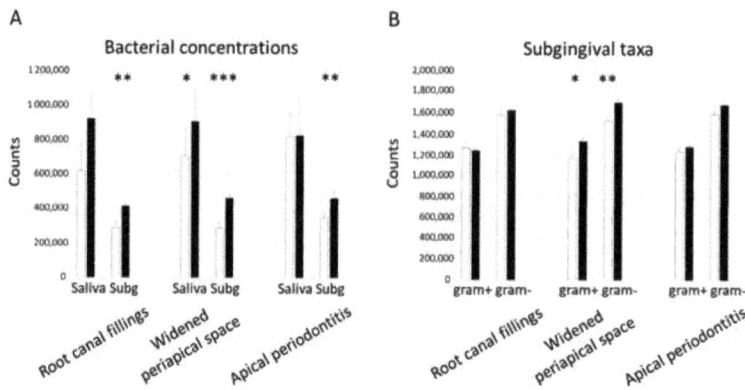

Figure 2. Saliva and subgingival bacteria according to endodontic findings. The patients were divided into groups according to the presence of root canal fillings, widened periapical spaces, and apical periodontitis. Salivary bacterial concentrations of *A. actinomycetemcomitans*, *P. gingivalis*, *P. intermedia*, and *T. forsythia* were determined by qPCR, and subgingival *A. actinomycetemcomitans*, *P. gingivalis*, *P. intermedia*, *P. endodontalis*, and *T. forsythia* by checkerboard DNA–DNA hybridization (A). This method was also used to examine subgingival 79 taxa, which were divided into Gram-positive ($n = 45$) and Gram-negative ($n = 34$) (B). The white columns depict the absence, and black columns presence of the endodontic finding. Means and standard errors are shown. The asterisks depict statistical significance between the groups defined by the *t*-test after logarithmic transformation: * $p < 0.05$, ** $p < 0.01$. *** $p < 0.001$.

The associations of antibody and bacterial levels with endodontic findings are presented in Table 2 for the whole population calculated by using linear and logistic regression models adjusted for age, sex, number of teeth, smoking, and status of marginal periodontitis. The estimates are presented for a 10-fold increase in the antibody or bacterial levels, number of root canal-treated teeth associated with saliva IgA and IgG against bacteria, and cross-reacting IgG. Among these, only saliva IgG against bacteria associated with the presence of root canal-treated teeth with an OR (95% CI) 2.52 (1.43–4.43).

Number of widened periapical spaces associated with saliva cross-reactive IgA and IgG, saliva IgG against bacteria, and subgingival bacteria in linear regression models. The presence of widened periapical spaces associated with saliva IgA and IgG against bacteria with ORs 2.09 (1.01–4.34) and 2.25 (1.40–3.61), respectively, and with cross-reacting IgG, 1.56 (1.22–1.99). Significant associations were also observed between the presence of widened periapical space and Gram-positive and Gram-negative subgingival bacteria with ORs 1.40 (1.02–1.92) and 1.45 (1.05–2.00). Number of teeth with apical periodontitis associated with saliva IgG against bacteria and cross-reacting IgG, which also presented significant ORs with the presence of apical periodontitis (2.90 (1.71–4.92) and 1.62 (1.24–2.11)).

A 3-category endodontic lesion score was designed for the severity of apical periodontitis. In addition, a 3-category endodontic treatment score was designed to investigate the contribution of treatment (root canal fillings) on the associations. The characteristics of the population are presented according to these scores in Table 3. Number of teeth, carious teeth, teeth with root canal fillings, and inadequate root canal fillings increased significantly with increasing scores. Also marginal periodontitis was more prevalent with high endodontic lesion ($p < 0.001$) or endodontic treatment ($p = 0.287$) score. Mean antibody levels in serum and saliva against specific antigens, as well as the saliva and subgingival bacterial levels according to these scores are presented in supplementary tables (Table S4 and S5). The association of the scores with the combined microbial biomarkers was analyzed by multinomial regression models for the $\log_{10}$-transforemed units (Figure 3). All measured parameters displayed positive trends with the increasing endodontic lesion score. Statistically significant associations (OR (95% CI)) with the highest endodontic scores were observed for saliva IgA (2.90 (1.01–8.33)) and IgG (4.91 (2.48–9.71)) against bacteria, saliva cross-reacting IgG (2.10 (1.48–2.97)), serum IgG against bacteria (4.66 (1.22–10.1)), subgingival species (1.15 (1.07–1.25)), and Gram-negative subgingival species (1.98 (1.16–3.37)). Regarding the treatment, only saliva IgG against bacteria, cross-reacting IgG, and serum IgA and IgG displayed increasing trends. Significant odds (OR (95%CI)) for untreated apical periodontitis were observed for saliva IgG against bacteria (5.32 (2.61–10.8)) and for cross-reacting IgG (2.04 (1.44–2.88)) (Figure 3).

The main results were reanalyzed in the subgroup of patients without marginal periodontitis ($n = 132$). There were no significant differences in the bacterial levels between groups divided according to the endodontic findings. Saliva IgG antibodies against bacteria and cross-reacting antibodies were higher in subjects with root canal fillings ($p = 0.003$ and 0.004), widened periapical spaces ($p = 0.008$ and 0.008), and apical periodontitis ($p = 0.012$ and 0.385). Both antibody levels increased in groups of patients with increasing endodontic scores (p for linear trend 0.009 and 0.020). The antibodies against bacteria (p for linear trend 0.007), but not the cross-reacting antibodies ($p = 0.569$), increased in patients with greater endodontic treatment scores. The associations of the saliva IgG class antibodies with endodontic lesion score and endodontic treatment score are presented in Table 4. Increasing trends were observed clearly only for saliva IgG against bacteria; the multivariate odds (OR (95% CI)) for having multiple teeth with apical periodontitis and for having teeth with untreated apical periodontitis were 3.45 (0.83–14.3) and 4.77 (1.05–21.7), respectively.

Table 2. Associations of endodontic findings with saliva and serum antibody levels and bacterial concentrations.

	Root Canal Fillings		Widened Periapical Space		Apical Periodontitis	
	Beta, p-Value	OR (95% CI), p	Beta, p-Value	OR (95% CI), p	Beta, p-Value	OR (95% CI), p
Saliva IgA against bacteria *	**0.096, 0.041**	2.162 (0.934–5.004), 0.072	0.062, 0.204	**2.090 (1.007–4.337), 0.048**	0.059, 0.235	1.995 (0.870–4.573), 0.103
Saliva IgG against bacteria *	**0.169, <0.001**	**2.519 (1.431–4.434), 0.001**	**0.138, 0.005**	**2.246 (1.397–3.611), 0.001**	**0.182, <0.001**	**2.904 (1.714–4.922), <0.001**
Serum IgA against bacteria *	0.031, 0.527	1.144 (0.516–2.539), 0.741	0.017, 0.738	1.513 (0.753–3.040), 0.245	0.037, 0.476	0.922 (0.421–2.018), 0.838
Serum IgG against bacteria *	0.010, 0.838	1.272 (0.443–3.656), 0.655	0.002, 0.963	2.048 (0.840–4.995), 0.115	0.083, 0.102	1.710 (0.615–4.754), 0.304
Saliva pathogen sum	0.012, 0.802	0.996 (0.932–1.064), 0.900	0.068, 0.163	1.046 (0.989–1.107), 0.117	0.079, 0.111	0.998 (0.936–1.064), 0.951
Subgingival pathogen sum	0.053, 0.273	0.991 (0.934–1.051), 0.760	0.086, 0.085	1.051 (0.999–1.105), 0.056	**0.098, 0.049**	1.047 (0.987–1.112), 0.127
45 gram-positive taxa	0.025, 0.603	0.754 (0.515–1.104), 0.147	**0.121, 0.014**	**1.395 (1.016–1.917), 0.040**	0.045, 0.375	1.096 (0.761–1.578), 0.622
33 gram-negative taxa	0.056, 0.237	0.945 (0.660–1.353), 0.757	**0.121, 0.014**	**1.446 (1.046–1.999), 0.026**	0.059, 0.238	1.249 (0.850–1.836), 0.257
Saliva cross-reactive IgA **	0.086, 0.067	1.248 (0.926–1.680), 0.146	**0.096, 0.049**	1.295 (0.995–1.685), 0.055	0.064, 0.196	1.327 (0.986–1.788), 0.062
Saliva cross-reactive IgG **	**0.128, 0.006**	1.240 (0.942–1.632), 0.125	**0.160, 0.001**	**1.555 (1.217–1.987), <0.001**	**0.159, 0.001**	**1.615 (1.237–2.108), <0.001**

The dependent variable in the linear regression was the number of findings and in the logistic regression the presence of findings. Adjusted for age, sex, marginal periodontitis (healthy, gingivitis, periodontitis), number of teeth, and smoking (never/ever). * Antibodies against *A. actinomycetemcomitans, P. gingivalis, P. intermedia, P. endodontalis*, and *T. forsythia*; ** Cross-reactive antibodies, antigens Pg-Rgp44, Aa-HSP60, and MAA-LDL.

Table 3. Characteristics of the population according to endodontic scores.

Character	Endodontic Lesion Score				Endodontic Treatment Score			
	Score I	Score II	Score III	P[1]	Score I	Score II	Score III	P[1]
	Mean (SD)				Mean (SD)			
Age (years)	63.3 (9.2)	63.1 (8.7)	63.7 (9.8)	0.924	63.3 (9.0)	64.3 (9.0)	62.5 (9.5)	0.578
BMI (kg/m^2)	27.8 (5.0)	27.8 (5.1)	27.8 (4.4)	0.990	27.7 (5.0)	27.9 (4.8)	28.2 (4.8)	0.852
Number of teeth	18.1 (10.5)	21.5 (7.3)	22.0 (6.7)	<0.001	19.7 (9.3)	23.2 (6.0)	20.5 (8.0)	0.031
	Mean (95% CI)				Mean (95% CI)			
Number of implants	0.17 (0.04–0.29)	0.10 (0.01–0.20)	0.12 (0.04–0.28)	0.696	0.15 (0.06–0.23)	0.14 (0.07–0.35)	0.02 (0.02–0.06)	0.546
Carious teeth	0.68 (0.52–0.84)	0.97 (0.75–1.18)	1.74 (1.20–2.27)	<0.001	0.83 (0.69–0.98)	1.24 (0.76–1.71)	1.82 (1.10–2.53)	<0.001
Root canal fillings	0.95 (0.73–1.17)	2.54 (2.26–2.82)	3.91 (3.21–4.61)	<0.001	1.82 (1.61–2.02)	4.65 (3.84–5.45)	1.91 (1.28–2.54)	<0.001
Inadequate root fillings	0.41 (0.29–0.52)	1.26 (1.10–1.42)	2.07 (1.64–2.51)	<0.001	0.88 (0.76–1.00)	2.33 (1.83–2.84)	1.05 (0.65–1.44)	<0.001
	N (%)			P[2]	N (%)			P[2]
N (%)	189 (41.7)	196 (43.3)	68 (15.0)		352 (77.7)	51 (11.3)	50 (11.0)	
Sex (males)	123 (65.1)	132 (67.3)	47 (69.1)	0.803	234 (66.5)	33 (64.7)	35 (70.0)	0.842
Smoking (ever)	92 (48.9)	112 (57.1)	35 (51.5)	0.265	190 (54.1)	23 (45.1)	26 (52.0)	0.478
Hypertension	122 (64.6)	123 (63.4)	41 (61.2)	0.885	226 (64.6)	30 (58.8)	30 (61.2)	0.683
Diabetes (type I/II)	39 (20.9)	47 (24.2)	14 (21.2)	0.711	78 (22.4)	11 (22.0)	11 (22.4)	0.998
Dyslipidemia	148 (78.3)	165 (85.5)	49 (73.1)	0.050	285 (81.7)	42 (84.0)	35 (70.0)	0.121
Marginal periodontitis	111 (58.7)	154 (78.6)	56 (82.4)	<0.001	244 (69.3)	37 (72.5)	40 (80.0)	0.287

[1] ANOVA; [2] Chi-square test; Endodontic lesion score: score I, no endodontic lesions; score II, patients with ≥1 widened periapical space and/or 1 tooth with apical periodontitis; and score III, patients with ≥2 teeth with apical periodontitis. Endodontic treatment score: score I, no endodontic lesions; score II, apical periodontitis only in teeth with root canal fillings; score III, apical periodontitis in teeth without root canal fillings.

Table 4. Association of saliva IgG class antibody levels with endodontic scores in the subpopulation free from marginal periodontitis.

		OR (95% CI), P-Value			
		Saliva IgG Against Bacteria *		Saliva Cross-Reacting IgG **	
		Univariate	Multivariate [1]	Univariate	Multivariate [1]
Endodontic lesion score	No endodontic lesions	1.0	1.0	1.0	1.0
	≥1 tooth with widened periapical space or apical periodontitis	2.92 (1.17–7.26), 0.022	2.67 (1.03–6.94), 0.044	2.06 (1.31–3.22), 0.002	1.97 (1.24–3.11), 0.004
	≥2 teeth with apical periodontitis	3.88 (0.99–15.5), 0.050	3.45 (0.83–14.3), 0.088	1.32 (0.65–2.69), 0.435	1.30 (0.64–2.62), 0.472
Endodontic treatment score	No endodontic lesions	1.0	1.0	1.0	1.0
	Apical periodontitis in teeth with root canal fillings	2.52 (0.70–9.06), 0.157	2.44 (0.66–9.06), 0.184	1.11 (0.60–2.03), 0.746	1.12 (0.60–2.08), 0.731
	Apical periodontitis in teeth without root canal fillings	5.88 (1.32–26.2), 0.020	4.77 (1.05–21.7), 0.043	1.43 (0.73–2.80), 0.297	1.39 (0.70–2.78), 0.351

[1] Adjusted for age, sex, and smoking (never/ever). Multinomial logistic regression. * Antibodies against *A. actinomycetemcomitans*, *P. gingivalis*, *P. intermedia*, *P. endodontalis*, and *T. forsythia*; ** Cross-reactive antibodies, antigens Pg-Rgp44, Aa-HSP60, and MAA-LDL.

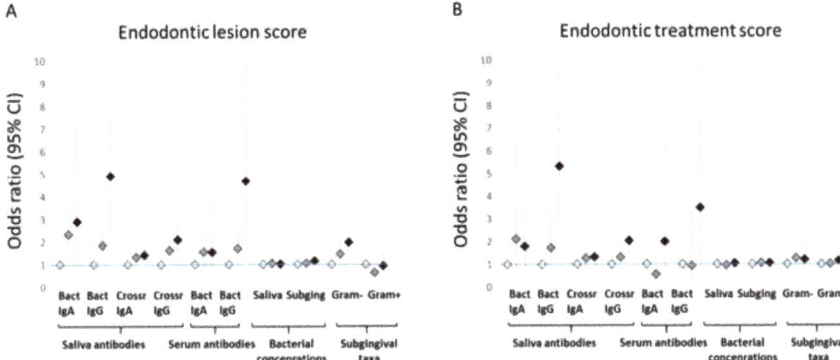

Figure 3. Associations of the antibody and bacterial levels with endodontic lesion score and endodontic treatment score. Endodontic lesion score (A): score I, no endodontic lesions; score II, patients with ≥1 widened periapical space and/or 1 tooth with apical periodontitis; and score III, patients with ≥2 teeth with apical periodontitis. Endodontic treatment score (B): score I, no endodontic lesions; score II, apical periodontitis only in teeth with root canal fillings; score III, apical periodontitis in teeth without root canal fillings. The associations were investigated by using multinomial regression models adjusted for age, sex, marginal periodontitis (healthy, gingivitis, periodontitis), number of teeth, and smoking (never/ever). The estimates for lowest (reference), middle, and highest scores are depicted with white, gray, and black diamonds, respectively.

4. Discussion

We showed that apical periodontitis is associated with elevated levels of saliva IgA and IgG and serum IgG against bacterial antigens and saliva cross-reacting IgG, which recognise both bacterial and host epitopes. The associations were independent of marginal periodontitis. The local antibody response may contribute to the systemic IgG levels, which associate with the severity of apical periodontitis and arise mainly from untreated apical infections. High salivary IgA was associated with the number of widened periapical spaces, most likely indicating early endodontic infection.

Elevated levels of salivary total IgG associated with endodontic findings including root canal treatments, widened periapical spaces and radiographically diagnosed apical periodontitis. Both the presence and number of endodontic findings were significantly associated with total salivary IgG levels. In the case of total salivary IgA, the presence of root canal fillings and the number of widened periapical spaces, but neither the presence nor the number of teeth with apical periodontitis, associated with higher antibody levels. In health, the saliva IgGs mainly derive from the circulation by transudation through the gingival crevice. They comprise less than 15 percent of the total salivary immunoglobulins, as the major salivary immunoglobulin is secretory IgA produced by the salivary glands in mucosal plasma cells [38,39]. However, high concentrations of IgG and IgA and smaller amounts of IgM and secretory IgA have been detected within the periapical granulomas, in periapical cysts, as well as in root canal exudates with periapically affected teeth [40]. In addition, the total IgG and IgA levels detected from the periapical exudate were shown to correlate with clinical findings of the infected teeth [41]. As the half-life of IgA-class antibodies is only a few days, they are considered to reflect either recent or repeated exposure to the pathogen, while IgG is more stable, thus indicating a past, and maybe chronic, infection. Widened periapical spaces reflect either symptomatic teeth with irreversible pulpitis or precursors for established AP in necrotic teeth [1]. Since all determined antibody levels and bacterial concentrations correlated with the endodontic score, our results support the suggestion that the widened periapical spaces are likely to reflect early endodontic lesions [20].

When antibody response was studied in more detail, it was observed that salivary IgG levels against all studied species (*A. actinomycetemcomitans, P. gingivalis, P. intermedia, P. endodontalis,* and *T. forsythia*) were significantly higher in the groups with endodontic findings. In addition, patients with widened periapical spaces had higher saliva IgA-antibodies against *P. endodontalis*. It is widely accepted that endodontic infections have a multimicrobial etiology [4], and several pathogens associated with marginal periodontitis, such as *P. intermedia*, *P. gingivalis*, *T. denticola* and *P. endodontalis*, are frequently detected in teeth with necrotic pulps [42–44]. As apical periodontitis is often restricted to the periapical tissues, it is not surprising that the amount of studied salivary and subgingival bacteria were not consistently associated with the endodontic findings. On the other hand, it is reported that in the case of combined endodontic-periodontal lesions, where apical periodontitis can be initiated either in the pulp or in the periodontium, the microbial profiles of apical lesions and periodontal pockets resemble each other [10]. In such cases, it is probable that bacteria enter the root canal from the periodontium via the apical foramen, dentinal tubules and accessory root canals [45].

Two major pathogens in marginal periodontitis, *A. actinomycetemcomitans* and *P. gingivalis*, express several virulence factors including *P. gingivalis*-specific gingipains degrading the extracellular matrix and bioactive peptides [46], as well as heat shock proteins (HSPs) produced by both species [47]. These proteins elicit strong antibody production and are also able to induce a variety of cross-reactive antibodies recognizing human epitopes such as HSPs and oxidized low-density lipoproteins (oxLDL). These cross-reactions are considered potential links between periodontitis and an increased risk of cardiovascular diseases [21]. The oxidation of LDL gives rise to various epitopes and a frequently used model of oxLDL include the immunodominant epitopes malondialdehyde (MDA) and malondialdehyde acetaldehyde (MAA). It is reported that the presence of antibodies binding to MDA-LDL is associated with both the progression of atherosclerosis and with the presence and severity of periodontitis [37,48–50]. A monoclonal IgM antibody to MDA-LDL recognizes *P. gingivalis* virulence factor gingipain (Rgp44) as an antigen [34] and *A. actinomycetemcomitans* heat shock protein 60 (Aa-HSP60) cross-reacts with MAA-LDL [35]. To our knowledge, this study is the first to show the association between apical periodontitis and salivary cross-reactive antibodies. Especially cross-reactive antibodies representing IgG-class were strongly associated with different endodontic conditions.

All measured parameters displayed positive trends with increasing number of endodontic findings as both the salivary IgA and IgG against bacterial antigens, as well as the cross-reacting IgG, were significantly associated with the highest endodontic score. In addition, the effect of endodontic treatment on antibody response was evident indicating that the levels of both saliva IgG against bacterial antigens and cross-reacting IgG were significantly higher in the patients with primary apical periodontitis compared to those who had apical periodontitis in teeth with root canal fillings. The aim of root canal treatment is to eradicate the biofilm from the infected root canal and prevent the recurrent infection. However, if the treatment is inadequately performed, some bacteria may survive and cause secondary infection. The microbiome of endodontically treated root canals consists of fewer bacterial species, and some of the species are more resilient to endodontic treatment [10]. This phenomenon may reflect to the levels of antibodies measured in this study.

The production of local IgGs is also enhanced in advanced marginal periodontitis by local plasma cells of the gingiva [51]. We repeated our main analyses in a subgroup of subjects without marginal periodontitis. Although the number of patients in this subgroup was low, the association between saliva IgG against bacterial antigens and primary apical periodontitis remained significant, suggesting further that IgG antibody response is independent of marginal periodontitis.

The main limitation of this study is that our study population consists of middle-aged and elderly participants, and thus the oral infections are very common. In addition, all participants had an initial indication for coronary angiography. Another restriction is the lack of intracanal bacterial samples; hence the bacterial analyses were only conducted from saliva and subgingival samples. Different methods were used for the detection of the antibody levels in serum and saliva, and not the same antibody panels were available. For instance, we did not have information on the serum cross-reactive antibodies, which will be an aim for future investigations. Also different methodologies were used for the bacterial analyses, since the subgingival samples were examined by checkerboard DNA–DNA hybridization and the saliva samples by qPCR.

Although apical periodontitis has been considered as a potential risk factor for systemic diseases such as coronary artery disease (CAD) [52], only a few studies have attempted to draw conclusions on the associations between apical periodontitis and systemic diseases. Evidence for the association between AP and CVDs, such as endothelial dysfunction [53], atherosclerosis [54], and coronary heart disease [55], has been reported in separate studies. However, recent systematic reviews suggest only modest participation of endodontic infection on the systemic levels of biomarkers and a moderate or low correlation between some systemic diseases and apical periodontitis [14,23,24,56]. In our recent study, we demonstrated a confounder-adjusted association between apical periodontitis and CAD [20]. In the present study, we showed that apical periodontitis may contribute to the levels of IgG in serum which link oral bacteria to CAD risk [31]. These serum antibodies have been repeatedly associated with prevalent and incident CVD as well as with subclinical atherosclerosis [57–60]. Also the saliva cross-reacting antibodies and immunoglobulins against bacterial antigens have been associated with increased risk for CAD [37].

Salivary immunoglobulins are potential biomarkers of oral infectious diseases, but the specific antigens should be selected carefully. This would be especially beneficial in the case of apical periodontitis, as the disease is often asymptomatic and remains undiagnosed. This study represents a limited set of antibodies against selected bacterial targets, and further research is needed to investigate the levels of antibodies against other bacterial species commonly found in infected root canals.

5. Conclusions

Our results suggest that the inflammatory condition caused by endodontic infections could be identified by the increased salivary IgG levels independently of marginal periodontitis. The levels of saliva IgG may have a small, but significant effect on the systemic levels of biomarkers, indicating the potential link between apical periodontitis and systemic diseases.

Supplementary Materials: The following are available online at http://www.mdpi.com/2077-0383/8/6/889/s1, Table S1: Bacterial species determined from subgingival plaque, Table S2: Saliva and serum antibody levels according to endodontic findings, Table S3: Saliva and subgingival bacterial levels according to endodontic findings, Table S4: Saliva and serum antibody levels according to endodontic scores, Table S5: Saliva and subgingival bacterial levels according to endodontic scores.

Author Contributions: Conceptualization, M.P. and P.J.P.; investigation—laboratory analyses, M.P., J.M.L., R.A., S.H., and P.J.P.; investigation—clinical examination, K.B., S.P., P.M., and J.S.; investigation—radiographic examination, J.M.L., K.B., S.P., A.S., P.M., and L.T.; formal analysis, M.P., A.S., and P.J.P.; writing—original draft preparation, M.P.; writing—review and editing, A.J., A.S., S.P., J.M.L., R.A., and P.J.P.; project administration, P.J.P; funding acquisition, S.P. and P.J.P.; supervision, P.J.P.

Funding: This research was funded by Academy of Finland [grant number 1266053 (P.J.P.), 1296541 (S.P.), and 1316777 (S.P.)], Paulo Foundation (P.J.P.), Finnish Dental Society Apollonia (P.J.P. and R.A.), University of Oulu Scholarship Foundation (R.A.) European Endodontic Society (P.J.P.), and Sigrid Juselius Foundation (P.J.P.).

Conflicts of Interest: The authors declare no conflicts of interest.

References

1. Carrotte, P. Endodontics: Part 3. Treatment of endodontic emergencies. *Br. Dent. J.* **2004**, *197*, 299–305. [CrossRef] [PubMed]
2. Pak, J.G.; Fayazi, S.; White, S.N. Prevalence of periapical radiolucency and root canal treatment: A systematic review of cross-sectional studies. *J. Endod.* **2012**, *38*, 1170–1176. [CrossRef] [PubMed]
3. Persoon, I.F.; Özok, A.R. Definitions and Epidemiology of Endodontic Infections. *Curr. Oral. Health Rep.* **2017**, *4*, 278–285. [CrossRef]
4. Siqueira, J.F., Jr.; Rôças, I.N. Distinctive features of the microbiota associated with different forms of apical periodontitis. *J. Oral. Microbiol.* **2009**, *1*. [CrossRef] [PubMed]
5. Hong, B.Y.; Lee, T.K.; Lim, S.M.; Chang, S.W.; Park, J.; Han, S.H.; Zhu, Q.; Safavi, K.E.; Fouad, A.F.; Kum, K.Y. Microbial analysis in primary and persistent endodontic infections by using pyrosequencing. *J. Endod.* **2013**, *39*, 1136–1140. [CrossRef] [PubMed]

6. Tzanetakis, G.N.; Azcarate-Peril, M.A.; Zachaki, S.; Panopoulos, P.; Kontakiotis, E.G.; Madianos, P.N.; Divaris, K. Comparison of Bacterial Community Composition of Primary and Persistent Endodontic Infections Using Pyrosequencing. *J. Endod.* **2015**, *41*, 1226–1233. [CrossRef] [PubMed]
7. Keskin, C.; Demiryürek, E.Ö.; Onuk, E.E. Pyrosequencing analysis of cryogenically ground samples from primary and secondary/persistent endodontic infections. *J. Endod.* **2017**, *43*, 1309–1316. [CrossRef] [PubMed]
8. Bouillaguet, S.; Manoil, D.; Girard, M.; Louis, J.; Gaïa, N.; Leo, S.; Schrenzel, J.; Lazarevic, V. Root Microbiota in Primary and Secondary Apical Periodontitis. *Front. Microbiol.* **2018**, *9*, 2374. [CrossRef] [PubMed]
9. Shin, J.M.; Luo, T.; Lee, K.H.; Guerreiro, D.; Botero, T.M.; McDonald, N.J.; Rickard, A.H. Deciphering Endodontic Microbial Communities by Next-generation Sequencing. *J. Endod.* **2018**, *44*, 1080–1087. [CrossRef]
10. Gomes, B.P.; Berber, V.B.; Kokaras, A.S.; Chen, T.; Paster, B.J. Microbiomes of Endodontic-Periodontal Lesions before and after Chemomechanical Preparation. *J. Endod.* **2015**, *4*, 1975–1984. [CrossRef] [PubMed]
11. Graunaite, I.; Lodiene, G.; Maciulskiene, V. Pathogenesis of apical periodontitis: A literature review. *J. Oral. Maxillofac. Res.* **2011**, *2*, e1. [CrossRef] [PubMed]
12. Hernández-Ríos, P.; Pussinen, P.J.; Vernal, R.; Hernández, M. Oxidative Stress in the Local and Systemic Events of Apical Periodontitis. *Front. Physiol.* **2017**, *1*, 869. [CrossRef] [PubMed]
13. Gomes, M.S.; Blattner, T.C.; Sant'Ana Filho, M.; Grecca, F.S.; Hugo, F.N.; Fouad, A.F.; Reynolds, M.A. Can apical periodontitis modify systemic levels of inflammatory markers? A systematic review and meta-analysis. *J. Endod.* **2013**, *39*, 1205–1217. [CrossRef] [PubMed]
14. Vidal, F.; Fontes, T.V.; Marques, T.V.; Gonçalves, L.S. Association between apical periodontitis lesions and plasmatic levels of C-reactive protein, interleukin 6 and fibrinogen in hypertensive patients. *Int. Endod. J.* **2016**, *49*, 1107–1115. [CrossRef] [PubMed]
15. Garrido, M.; Cárdenas, A.M.; Astorga, J.; Quinlan, F.; Valdés, M.; Chaparro, A.; Carvajal, P.; Pussinen, P.; Huamán-Chipana, P.; Jalil, J.E.; et al. Elevated Systemic Inflammatory Burden and Cardiovascular Risk in Young Adults with Endodontic Apical Lesions. *J. Endod.* **2019**, *45*, 111–115. [CrossRef] [PubMed]
16. Greening, A.B.; Schonfeld, S.E. Apical lesions contain elevated immunoglobulin G levels. *J. Endod.* **1980**, *12*, 867–869. [CrossRef]
17. Johannessen, A.C.; Nilsen, R.; Skaug, N. Deposits of immunoglobulins and complement factor C3 in human dental periapical inflammatory lesions. *Scand. J. Dent. Res.* **1983**, *91*, 191–199. [CrossRef]
18. Keudell, K.; Powel, G.; Berry, H. A review of microbial and immunologic aspects of endodontics. *J. Oral. Pathol. Med.* **1981**, *36*, 39–43.
19. Torres, J.O.C.; Torabinejad, M.; Matiz, R.A.R.; Mantilla, E.G. Presence of secretory IgA in human periapical lesions. *J. Endod.* **1994**, *20*, 87–89. [CrossRef]
20. Liljestrand, J.M.; Mäntylä, P.; Paju, S.; Buhlin, K.; Kopra, K.A.; Persson, G.R.; Hernandez, M.; Nieminen, M.S.; Sinisalo, J.; Tjäderhane, L.; et al. Association of Endodontic Lesions with Coronary Artery Disease. *J. Dent. Res.* **2016**, *95*, 1358–1365. [CrossRef]
21. Pietiäinen, M.; Liljestrand, J.M.; Kopra, E.; Pussinen, P.J. Mediators between oral dysbiosis and cardiovascular diseases. *Eur. J. Oral. Sci.* **2018**, *126* (Suppl. 1), 26–36. [CrossRef] [PubMed]
22. Lockhart, P.B.; Bolger, A.F.; Papapanou, P.N.; Osinbowale, O.; Trevisan, M.; Levison, M.E.; Taubert, K.A.; Newburger, J.W.; Gornik, H.L.; Gewitz, M.H.; et al. Periodontal disease and atherosclerotic vascular disease: Does the evidence support an independent association? A scientific statement from the American Heart Association. *Circulation* **2012**, *125*, 2520–2544. [CrossRef] [PubMed]
23. Khalighinejad, N.; Aminoshariae, M.R.; Aminoshariae, A.; Kulild, J.C.; Mickel, A.; Fouad, A.F. Association between systemic diseases and apical periodontitis. *J. Endod.* **2016**, *42*, 1427–1434. [CrossRef] [PubMed]
24. Berlin-Broner, Y.; Febbraio, M.; Levin, L. Association between apical periodontitis and cardiovascular diseases: A systematic review of the literature. *Int. Endod. J.* **2017**, *50*, 847–859. [CrossRef] [PubMed]
25. Vaara, S.; Nieminen, M.S.; Lokki, M.L.; Perola, M.; Pussinen, P.J.; Allonen, J.; Parkkonen, O.; Sinisalo, J. Cohort Profile: The Corogene study. *Int. J. Epidemiol.* **2012**, *41*, 1265–1271. [CrossRef] [PubMed]
26. Buhlin, K.; Mäntylä, P.; Paju, S.; Peltola, J.S.; Nieminen, M.S.; Sinisalo, J.; Pussinen, P.J. Periodontitis is associated with angiographically verified coronary artery disease. *J. Clin. Periodontol.* **2011**, *38*, 1007–1014. [CrossRef] [PubMed]

27. Liljestrand, J.M.; Paju, S.; Buhlin, K.; Persson, G.R.; Sarna, S.; Nieminen, M.S.; Sinisalo, J.; Mäntylä, P.; Pussinen, P.J. Lipopolysaccharide, a possible molecular mediator between periodontitis and coronary artery disease. *J. Clin. Periodontol.* **2017**, *44*, 784–792. [CrossRef]
28. Mäntylä, P.; Buhlin, K.; Paju, S.; Persson, G.R.; Nieminen, M.S.; Sinisalo, J.; Pussinen, P.J. Subgingival *Aggregatibacter actinomycetemcomitans* associates with the risk of coronary artery disease. *J. Clin. Periodontol.* **2013**, *40*, 583–590. [CrossRef]
29. Socransky, S.S.; Haffajee, A.D.; Smith, C.; Martin, L.; Haffajee, J.A.; Uzel, N.G.; Goodson, J.M. Use of checkerboard DNA-DNA hybridization to study complex microbial ecosystems. *Oral. Microbiol. Immunol.* **2004**, *19*, 352–362. [CrossRef]
30. Hyvärinen, K.; Mäntylä, P.; Buhlin, K.; Paju, S.; Nieminen, M.S.; Sinisalo, J.; Pussinen, P.J. A common periodontal pathogen has an adverse association with both acute and stable coronary artery disease. *Atherosclerosis* **2012**, *223*, 478–484. [CrossRef]
31. Liljestrand, J.M.; Paju, S.; Pietiäinen, M.; Buhlin, K.; Persson, G.R.; Nieminen, M.S.; Sinisalo, J.; Mäntylä, P.; Pussinen, P.J. Immunologic burden links periodontitis to acute coronary syndrome. *Atherosclerosis* **2018**, *268*, 177–184. [CrossRef] [PubMed]
32. Pussinen, P.J.; Könönen, E.; Paju, S.; Hyvärinen, K.; Gursoy, U.K.; Huumonen, S.; Knuuttila, M.; Suominen, A.L. Periodontal pathogen carriage, rather than periodontitis, determines the serum antibody levels. *J. Clin. Periodontol.* **2011**, *38*, 405–411. [CrossRef] [PubMed]
33. Hörkkö, S.; Bird, D.A.; Miller, E.; Itabe, H.; Leitinger, N.; Subbanagounder, G.; Berliner, J.A.; Friedman, P.; Dennis, E.A.; Curtiss, L.K.; et al. Monoclonal autoantibodies specific for oxidized phospholipids or oxidized phospholipid-protein adducts inhibit macrophage uptake of oxidized low-density lipoproteins. *J. Clin. Investig.* **1999**, *103*, 117–128. [CrossRef] [PubMed]
34. Turunen, S.P.; Kummu, O.; Harila, K.; Veneskoski, M.; Soliymani, R.; Baumann, M.; Pussinen, P.J.; Hörkkö, S. Recognition of *Porphyromonas gingivalis* gingipain epitopes by natural IgM binding to malondialdehyde modified low-density lipoprotein. *PLoS ONE* **2012**, *7*, e34910. [CrossRef]
35. Wang, C.; Kankaanpää, J.; Kummu, O.; Turunen, S.P.; Akhi, R.; Bergmann, U.; Pussinen, P.; Remes, A.M.; Hörkkö, S. Characterization of a natural mouse monoclonal antibody recognizing epitopes shared by oxidized lowdensity lipoprotein and chaperonin 60 of *Aggregatibacter actinomycetemcomitans*. *Immunol. Res.* **2016**, *64*, 699–710. [CrossRef] [PubMed]
36. Karvonen, J.; Päivänsalo, M.; Kesäniemi, Y.A.; Hörkkö, S. Immunoglobulin M type of autoantibodies to oxidized low-density lipoprotein has an inverse relation to carotid artery atherosclerosis. *Circulation* **2003**, *108*, 2107–2112. [CrossRef]
37. Akhi, R.; Wang, C.; Nissinen, A.E.; Kankaanpää, J.; Bloigu, R.; Paju, S.; Mäntylä, P.; Buhlin, K.; Sinisalo, J.; Pussinen, P.J.; et al. Salivary IgA to MAA-LDL and Oral Pathogens Are Linked to Coronary Disease. *J. Dent. Res.* **2019**, *98*, 296–303. [CrossRef]
38. Gao, X.; Jiang, S.; Koh, D.; Hsu, C.Y. Salivary biomarkers for dental caries. *Periodontology 2000* **2016**, *70*, 128–141. [CrossRef]
39. Brandtzaeg, P. Secretory immunity with special reference to the oral cavity. *J. Oral. Microbiol.* **2013**, *5*, 20401. [CrossRef]
40. Marton, I.J.; Kiss, C. Protective and destructive immune reactions in apical periodontitis. *Oral. Microbiol. Immunol.* **2000**, *15*, 139–150. [CrossRef]
41. Matsuo, T.; Nakanishi, T.; Ebisu, S. Immunoglobulins in periapical exudates of infected root canals: Correlation with the clinical findings of the involved teeth. *Endod. Dent. Traumatol.* **1995**, *11*, 95–99. [CrossRef]
42. Gomes, B.P.; Jacinto, R.C.; Pinheiro, E.T.; Sousa, E.L.; Zaia, A.A.; Ferraz, C.C.; Souza-Filho, F.J. *Porphyromonas gingivalis, Porphyromonas endodontalis, Prevotella intermedia* and *Prevotella nigrescens* in endodontic lesions detected by culture and by PCR. *Oral. Microbiol. Immunol.* **2005**, *20*, 211–215. [CrossRef] [PubMed]
43. Tomazinho, L.F.; Avila-Campos, M.J. Detection of *Porphyromonas gingivalis, Porphyromonas endodontalis, Prevotella intermedia,* and *Prevotella nigrescens* in chronic endodontic infection. *Oral Surg. Oral Med. Oral Pathol. Oral Radiol. Endod.* **2007**, *103*, 285–288. [CrossRef] [PubMed]
44. Martinho, F.C.; Chiesa, W.M.; Leite, F.R.; Cirelli, J.A.; Gomes, B.P. Antigenic activity of bacterial endodontic contents from primary root canal infection with periapical lesions against macrophage in the release of interleukin-1beta and tumor necrosis factor alpha. *J. Endod.* **2010**, *36*, 1467–1474. [CrossRef]

45. Solomon, C.; Chalfin, H.; Kellert, M.; Weseley, P. The endodontic-periodontal lesion: A rational approach to treatment. *J. Am. Dent. Assoc.* **1995**, *126*, 473–479. [CrossRef] [PubMed]
46. Potempa, J.; Pike, R.; Travis, J. Titration and mapping of the active site of cysteine proteinases from *Porphyromonas gingivalis* (gingipains) using peptidyl chloromethanes. *Biol. Chem.* **1997**, *378*, 223–230. [CrossRef]
47. Ford, P.J.; Gemmell, E.; Hamlet, S.M.; Hasan, A.; Walker, P.J.; West, M.J.; Cullinan, M.P.; Seymour, G.J. Cross-reactivity of GroEL antibodies with human heat shock protein 60 and quantification of pathogens in atherosclerosis. *Oral. Microbiol. Immunol.* **2005**, *20*, 296–302. [CrossRef]
48. Montebugnoli, L.; Servidio, D.; Miaton, R.A.; Prati, C.; Tricoci, P.; Melloni, C.; Melandri, G. Periodontal health improves systemic inflammatory and haemostatic status in subjects with coronary heart disease. *J. Clin. Periodontol.* **2005**, *32*, 188–192. [CrossRef]
49. Monteiro, A.M.; Jardini, M.A.; Alves, S.; Giampaoli, V.; Aubin, E.C.; Figueiredo Neto, A.M.; Gidlund, M. Cardiovascular disease parameters in periodontitis. *J. Periodontol.* **2009**, *80*, 378–388. [CrossRef]
50. Buhlin, K.; Holmer, J.; Gustafsson, A.; Hörkkö, S.; Pockley, A.G.; Johansson, A.; Paju, S.; Klinge, B.; Pussinen, P.J. Association of periodontitis with persistent, pro-atherogenic antibody responses. *J. Clin. Periodontol.* **2015**, *42*, 1006–1014. [CrossRef]
51. Russell, M.W.; Hajishengallis, G.; Childers, N.K.; Michalek, S.M. Secretory Immunity in Defense against Cariogenic Mutans Streptococci. *Caries Res.* **1999**, *33*, 4–15. [CrossRef] [PubMed]
52. Mattila, K.J.; Nieminen, M.S.; Valtonen, V.V.; Rasi, V.P.; Kesäniemi, Y.A.; Syrjälä, S.L.; Jungell, P.S.; Isoluoma, M.; Hietaniemi, K.; Jokinen, M.J. Association between dental health and acute myocardial infarction. *BMJ* **1989**, *298*, 779–781. [CrossRef] [PubMed]
53. Cotti, E.; Dessi, C.; Piras, A.; Flore, G.; Deidda, M.; Madeddu, C.; Zedda, A.; Longu, G.; Mercuro, G. Association of endodontic infection with detection of an initial lesion to the cardiovascular system. *J. Endod.* **2011**, *37*, 1624–1629. [CrossRef] [PubMed]
54. Petersen, J.; Glaßl, E.M.; Nasseri, P.; Crismani, A.; Luger, A.K.; Schoenherr, E.; Bertl, K.; Glodny, B. The association of chronic apical periodontitis and endodontic therapy with atherosclerosis. *Clin. Oral Investig.* **2014**, *18*, 1813–1823. [CrossRef] [PubMed]
55. Pasqualini, D.; Bergandi, L.; Palumbo, L.; Borraccino, A.; Dambra, V.; Alovisi, M.; Migliaretti, G.; Ferraro, G.; Ghigo, D.; Bergerone, S.; et al. Association among oral health, apical periodontitis, CD14 polymorphisms, and coronary heart disease in middle-aged adults. *J. Endod.* **2012**, *38*, 1570–1577. [CrossRef] [PubMed]
56. Aminoshariae, A.; Kulild, J.C.; Fouad, A.F. The Impact of Endodontic Infections on the Pathogenesis of Cardiovascular Disease(s): A Systematic Review with Meta-analysis Using GRADE. *J. Endod.* **2018**, *44*, 1361–1366.e3. [CrossRef] [PubMed]
57. Pussinen, P.J.; Jousilahti, P.; Alfthan, G.; Palosuo, T.; Asikainen, S.; Salomaa, V. Antibodies to periodontal pathogens are associated with coronary heart disease. *Arterioscler. Thromb. Vasc. Biol.* **2003**, *23*, 1250–1254. [CrossRef]
58. Pussinen, P.J.; Alfthan, G.; Rissanen, H.; Reunanen, A.; Asikainen, S.; Knekt, P. Antibodies to periodontal pathogens and stroke risk. *Stroke* **2004**, *35*, 2020–2023. [CrossRef]
59. Pussinen, P.J.; Nyyssönen, K.; Alfthan, G.; Salonen, R.; Laukkanen, J.A.; Salonen, J.T. Serum antibody levels to *Actinobacillus actinomycetemcomitans* predict the risk for coronary heart disease. *Arterioscler. Thromb. Vasc. Biol.* **2005**, *25*, 833–838. [CrossRef]
60. Beck, J.D.; Eke, P.; Heiss, G.; Madianos, P.; Couper, D.; Lin, D.; Moss, K.; Elter, J.; Offenbacher, S. Periodontal disease and coronary heart disease: A reappraisal of the exposure. *Circulation* **2005**, *112*, 19–24. [CrossRef]

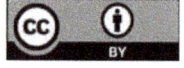 © 2019 by the authors. Licensee MDPI, Basel, Switzerland. This article is an open access article distributed under the terms and conditions of the Creative Commons Attribution (CC BY) license (http://creativecommons.org/licenses/by/4.0/).

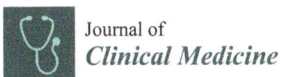

Review

Importance of Virulence Factors for the Persistence of Oral Bacteria in the Inflamed Gingival Crevice and in the Pathogenesis of Periodontal Disease

Gunnar Dahlen *, Amina Basic and Johan Bylund

Department of Oral Microbiology and Immunology, Institute of Odontology, Sahlgrenska Academy, University of Gothenburg, SE-40530 Gothenburg, Sweden
* Correspondence: dahlen@odontologi.gu.se; Tel.: +46-317-863-262

Received: 16 August 2019; Accepted: 22 August 2019; Published: 29 August 2019

Abstract: Periodontitis is a chronic inflammation that develops due to a destructive tissue response to prolonged inflammation and a disturbed homeostasis (dysbiosis) in the interplay between the microorganisms of the dental biofilm and the host. The infectious nature of the microbes associated with periodontitis is unclear, as is the role of specific bacterial species and virulence factors that interfere with the host defense and tissue repair. This review highlights the impact of classical virulence factors, such as exotoxins, endotoxins, fimbriae and capsule, but also aims to emphasize the often-neglected cascade of metabolic products (e.g., those generated by anaerobic and proteolytic metabolism) that are produced by the bacterial phenotypes that survive and thrive in deep, inflamed periodontal pockets. This metabolic activity of the microbes aggravates the inflammatory response from a low-grade physiologic (homeostatic) inflammation (i.e., gingivitis) into more destructive or tissue remodeling processes in periodontitis. That bacteria associated with periodontitis are linked with a number of systemic diseases of importance in clinical medicine is highlighted and exemplified with rheumatoid arthritis, The unclear significance of a number of potential "virulence factors" that contribute to the pathogenicity of specific bacterial species in the complex biofilm–host interaction clinically is discussed in this review.

Keywords: periodontal disease; host response; infection; inflammation; oral microbiota; virulence factors; metabolites

1. Introduction

Periodontal diseases affect the supporting tissues of teeth. The most common, gingivitis and periodontitis, are inflammatory diseases that are induced and maintained by the polymicrobial biofilm (dental plaque) that are formed on teeth in the absence of daily oral hygiene procedures. While gingivitis is a reversible inflammatory response without loss of bone support, periodontitis includes the destruction of the periodontal attachment and the alveolar bone. Peri-implantitis is the term used for a similar inflammatory reaction as periodontitis, but around dental implants, also here including the loss of bone support [1].

Periodontitis is the result of a complex interplay between microorganisms of the dental biofilm and the host. The role of specific microorganisms and their products in the disease initiation and propagation is still unclear [2,3]. The severity of the periodontal disease also depends on environmental (e.g., smoking) and host risk factors (for example genetic susceptibility) [4]. Lately, numerous studies have shown associations between periodontal disease and a number of systemic diseases, such as cardiovascular disease, diabetes mellitus, Alzheimer's disease, and rheumatoid arthritis [5]. This has intensified the research on the role of the microorganisms and their virulence factors in periodontitis. The purpose of this review is to high-light the complexity of the host-microbe relationship in periodontitis as well as the capacity of ordinary low virulent oral commensals to adapt and survive in the periodontal pocket, and to become infectious and contribute to systemic effects on the host.

2. The Role of Micro-organisms in Periodontitis—A Historical Perspective

The paradigm that dental plaque was the cause of gingivitis was established in the "gingivitis in man study" [6], where, in an experimental approach, a group of volunteers abstained from oral hygiene procedures resulting in plaque accumulation and gingivitis development. When oral hygiene procedures were reinstalled, the gingivitis was resolved within a week. The interpretation that followed was that the dental plaque induced the gingival inflammation and, if left untreated, this would inevitably lead to periodontitis [3]. Plaque was thought to cause periodontitis, and therefore plaque control became the cornerstone in the treatment of periodontal disease, and still is. Since the periodontitis distribution in the population was skewed, focus was next directed to specific bacteria, present in the dental biofilm of gingival/periodontal pockets and were more or less associated with periodontitis. Specific microorganisms, termed "putative periodontal pathogens", were hypothesized to be responsible for gingival tissue breakdown and the disease progression [7,8]. Even if Koch's postulate was found to be inadequate to apply to complex diseases like periodontitis, additional criteria for the elucidation of pathogens capable of causing periodontitis were suggested [9]. This bacteria-centered view of the disease led to the concept of an infectious nature of periodontitis, where treatment was aimed at eliminating putative pathogens e.g., with antibiotics [10].

It soon became clear that bacteria in the polymicrobial biofilm were necessary but not sufficient to explain why some individuals developed periodontitis while others did not, despite a similar composition of the subgingival microbiota. The existence of refractory cases that responded poorly to treatment and in which the disease continued to progress despite comprehensive periodontal treatment directed the focus towards the host and the inflammatory response—the disease susceptibility model [3,11,12]. This host-centered approach in search for high-risk groups and individuals discovered that diabetes patients or smokers were overrepresented among those with severe periodontitis [13,14]. The focus was on the host response and search for genetic grounds became intensive based on family pattern and twin studies of periodontitis [15,16]. The general epidemiological pattern, comprising of approximately 10–12% of the populations worldwide, irrespective of hygiene level and access to dental treatment, suffering from severe periodontitis with the risk of tooth loss [17] indicates that subgroups with genetic susceptibility for severe periodontitis exist in all populations. In a recent review it was concluded that up to one third of the variance of periodontitis is due to genetic factors [16]. The search for specific genes or gene polymorphism to explain the genetic role in periodontitis have so far been only moderately successful but the heritability of the disease is extremely complex and likely also influenced by epigenetic mechanisms [18,19].

While bacteria have a clear role in the periodontal disease aetiology, the relationship to other microorganisms, such as yeasts, is more uncertain [20]. Herpesviruses and Epstein-Barr virus, on the other hand, have been more strongly implicated in periodontitis and a link has also been suggested between periodontal herpesviruses and systemic diseases [21].

Nowadays periodontitis is described as an inflammatory disease induced and maintained by the polymicrobial biofilm formed on teeth, based on the polymicrobial synergy and dysbiosis hypothesis [22–24]. This hypothesis implies that the balance (homeostasis) between the microorganisms in the dental biofilm and the host response is disrupted due to fluctuations and burst of activity of the microorganisms or due to an imbalanced host response. This imbalanced condition in which the normal microbiome structure is disturbed is termed dysbiosis [24]. The magnitude of the inflammatory response is host related (susceptibility) and host related factors are responsible for the disease progression. The role of the classic, putative periodontal pathogens is still unclear and the infectious nature of the disease has been depreciated [23–25]. However, the enormous complexity and variability that takes place within the dental biofilm community and the similar complexity and variability in the inflammatory response is challenging. The role of the microorganisms in periodontitis is poorly understood and the many hypothesis launched are still hypotheses.

3. "Putative Periodontal Pathogens"

Aggregatibacter actinomycetemcomitans (previously *Actinobacillus actinomycetemcomitans*) was discovered to be closely related to localized forms of periodontal disease in young individuals. This discovery made it plausible that some microorganisms were more important for periodontal disease development than others and such microorganisms were termed "putative periodontal pathogens" [25,26]. Later, Socransky et al. [27] grouped three species (*Porphyromonas gingivalis*, *Tannerella forsythia* and *Treponema denticola*) to the so-called red complex, which was statistically strongly associated with periodontitis (Table 1). Another group including species such as *Prevotella intermedia*, *Fusobacterium nucleatum*, *Campylobacter rectus* and *Campylobacter gracilis* were associated with periodontitis to a milder degree and these were termed the orange complex [27]. Notably, most of these putative periodontopathogens are Gram-negative, strictly anaerobic species (except for *A. acinomyctemcomitans*), as well as proteolytic and thus well adapted to the inflamed periodontal pocket (Table 1). Occasional Gram-positive species, e.g., *Parvimonas micra* (formerly *Peptostreptococcus micros*) were included in the orange complex [27].

While some species, such as *A. actinomyctemcomitans* and *P. gingivalis*, are extremely well studied and described in several recent reviews, e.g., [28–30], phenotypical characterization of other bacterial species is more limited. Spirochetes are seriously underestimated, although they have been known to predominate the deep periodontal pocket from microscopic studies in the 1970s [31]. Studies using molecular biology methods have disclosed a number of unculturable *Treponema* genotypes, but their phenotypic characteristics are largely unknown [32,33].

It should also be noted that the concept of "species" is a man-made distinction and most species can be further specified into genotypic and/or phenotypic subtypes based on defined criteria. Clearly certain subtypes are more associated to oral infections than others, but unfortunately, the identification of bacterial species to a subtype level is rare in clinical oral microbiology studies. The best-known example of a specific bacterial subtype with implications for periodontal disease is the JP2 genotype of *A. actinomycetemcomitans*, which is a high virulent clone (high toxic clone) strongly associated with severe periodontal breakdown in young individuals of West African populations [34].

The list of "putative periodontal pathogens", or bacterial species associated to periodontitis, has gradually expanded and included 17 different species in a recent review [35]. Along with the use of more sensitive detection methods such as NGS (Next generation sequencing) the number periodontitis associated microorganisms have expanded further but their role in the pathogenesis of periodontitis remains elusive [36,37]. It is possible that certain microorganisms are more important for periodontal disease progression than others, but that can only be ruled out in prospective longitudinal studies over years without intervention, and very few such studies have been conducted [38].

Table 1. Important characteristics for eight "putative periodontal pathogens" as described by Socransky et al. (1998) in colored complexes (as indicated in the table by the red and orange color) associated with periodontitis. *A. actinomycetemcomitans* (serotype b) did not fit into any of the complexes and is colored grey in the table.

"Putative Periodontal Pathogens"	Gram Stain	Main Metabolic Trait	Motility	Proteolytic Activity	Carbohydrate Fermentation	Major end Products	Factors of Significance	Subtyping
Aggregatibacter actinomycetemcomitans	Gramneg	Facultative anaerobic	No	Weak	Glycolytic	Lactic acid, Succinic acid, Acetic acid, Propionic acid	Leukotoxin Cytodescen-ding (Cdt) toxin	Serotypes a-e, Non-serotypable isolates are frequent Specific genotypes (JP2)
Porphyromonas gingivalis	Gramneg	Anaerobic	No	Strong	Asaccharolytic	NH_3 H_2S Phenylacetic acid Indole	Gingipains (RgpA and Kgp)	FimA genotypes: I-V Arg-specific RgpA: A-C Lys-specific Kgp: I and II Capsular subtypes: K1-K6
Tannerella forsythia	Gramneg	Anaerobic	No	Strong	Weak glycolytic	H_2S (weak) Acetic acid Propionic acid	Trypsin-like and PrtH proteases	Variations in the leucine-rich repeat BspA protein are existing but no subtyping is presented
Treponema denticola	Gramneg	Anaerobic	Strong	Strong	Weak glycolytic	H_2S (strong)	Spirochetes (spiral shaped)	Seven oral Treponema species identified but no subtyping is known Hundreds of spirochetal genotypes (OTU's) found
Prevotella intermedia/nigrescens	Gramneg	Anaerobic	No	Strong	Glycolytic	NH_3 H_2S Succinic acid Acetic	Indole	Capsule is produced but no subtyping is known
Fusobacterium nucleatum	Gramneg	Anaerobic	No	Strong	Glycolytic	NH_3 H2S (strong) Butyric acid	Fusiform Morphology (threadlike)	Three subspecies reported variation in the outer-membrane structure
Campylobacter rectus/gracilis	Gramneg	Microaerophilic	weak	Weak	Asaccharolytic	H_2S Succinic acid	Nd	not known
Parvimonas micra	Grampos	Anaerobic	No	Strong	Glycolytic	NH_3 H_2S (weak), Acetic acid	Nd	not known

4. Periodontitis—An Inflammatory Disease or an Infectious Disease?

Inflammation is a host tissue response to an assault commonly triggered by microorganisms (or other stimuli such as chemicals, radiation and trauma) and their products (metabolites, endotoxins) released from them. Clinically, inflammation often relates to some kind of pathology, but it is important to remember that inflammatory reactions are absolutely critical for our well-being and the process has evolved to provide rapid and early protection. We likely experience thousands of small clinically 'invisible' inflammatory reactions along the mucosal membranes every day as a result of various assaults involving microorganisms, without considering these inflammatory responses as infections (or even disease). These cases could not be considered pathologic and represent situations where the inflammatory response is physiologic and provide early protection from potentially dangerous events (see below).

There are many definitions of infection, most of them aimed at primary pathogens and specific infections, while it is more controversial to find a definition that fits to infections involving commensals [39]. In line with the "damage-response framework" [39], which can be applied to various oral infections, the term infection can be defined as "the process in which pathogenic organisms (ambionts) invade the tissues or organs of the body and cause injury (damage) followed by reactive phenomena" according to Dorland´s Medical Dictionary [40,41]. The critical issue here is invasion (further discussed below) and ordinary commensals are not part of any infection as long as they are colonizing (present) on the external side of the epithelial lining (barrier). That is a 'normal' condition. This means that in a state of commensalism and colonization (such as the subgingival dental plaque in health or gingivitis) a homeostatic balance between the microbiota and the host response (a homeostatic inflammation) is created, according to Lamont et al. [23]. This controlled immune-inflammatory state where the inflammatory response of the host causes no apparent damage should not be considered as pathological but rather as a normal response (a physiological inflammation). Thus, gingival inflammation as a response to the dental biofilm is a state of normality developed through the evolution and present in almost 100% of adults of all populations worldwide [24,42].

Infection occurs when the virulence, the number, and the exposed time supersede the local and general host's defense, which leads to a pathological reaction in the host's tissues [43]. Virulence is the relative ability of a microorganism to cause disease and consequently, virulence is a microbial property that can only be expressed in a susceptible host. Hence, virulence is not an independent microbial property, because it cannot be defined independently of a host [39]. In that perspective all bacteria in the dental biofilm may contribute to the host response and it is not meaningful to distinguish pathogenic microbes from non-pathogenic at that stage (gingivitis). The dental biofilm is the natural habit for these microorganisms and the change in microbial composition that occurs over time may just be a consequence of the changing environment brought about by the host (inflammatory) response. This implies that bacterial species that are better adapted to the changing environment (deeper pocket, anaerobiosis, mechanical retention, alkaline environment, and increased exudate flow with an abundance of serum proteins, complement factors, neutrophils, lysozyme) will thrive and thereby increasingly (or at least consistently) fuel the inflammatory response. This may occur without bacterial invasion and also without necessarily causing any apparent damage. Therefore, gingivitis is not defined as an infection.

In certain periodontal conditions aside from chronic periodontitis, the case for an infectious nature of the problem is strong, e.g., exacerbations and abscess formation due to trauma or blockage of drainage by, e.g., calculus, fillings, or prosthesis. Periodontal infections resemble other dentoalveolar infections regarding their microbial composition and progression [44]. They are endogenic polymicrobial, predominantly anaerobic infections that are characterized by a destroyed internal regulation in the biofilm community with increased activity and growth of bacteria (burst) originating from the dental biofilm. In addition, periodontal infections usually feature bacterial invasion which requires detachment from the plaque. One other condition where bacterial invasion is rather obvious is peri-implantitis which is an endogenic polymicrobial anaerobic infection where the bacteria originate from the biofilm on the implant surface and with a microbiota which resembles that of the periodontal pocket [45]. Due to the anatomical difference from teeth and lack of an intact epithelial barrier, bacterial invasion can be facilitated in peri-implantitis. Clinically visible pus formation and increased number of neutrophils found in biopsies support the view of peri-implantitis as an infectious process [46].

In these conditions mentioned above (periodontal infections), the infections are polymicrobial and although some bacterial species are more frequently found (and may even play an important role), it is not possible to exclude any of the microorganisms from taking part in the "infection" and to solely act as innocent bystanders [2]. Numerous studies have been performed to explain virulence mechanisms in vitro but in accordance with the above definition of virulence this cannot be fully evaluated for various microorganisms independently of a host. However, experimental infections in animals have clearly shown that mixed infections are more infectious than mono-infections, and have also emphasized the importance of anaerobes without the necessity to include "putative pathogens" in such infections [47].

In contrast to periodontal infections, chronic periodontitis is a pathological inflammatory disease, as a response to prolonged (months, years) exposure to, and not infected by a polymicrobial community in the gingival/periodontal pocket. The tissue responses involve alternating destructive phases and repair or healing phases, but with a net loss of attachment and bone. The microorganisms are necessary components but not sufficient to explain the tissue damage. In view of the "damage–response framework" as discussed earlier, both the host and microbes contribute to pathogenesis. As mentioned, the role of specific microorganisms and certain virulence mechanisms in triggering this pathologic inflammation remain unclear. Most factors that are commonly discussed in terms of "virulence factors" among the putative periodontal pathogens should rather be termed "survival factors" since they do not necessarily constitute factors for pathogenicity and damage but for the living, growth and survival of the bacteria in deep, inflamed periodontal pockets.

5. Factors that Promote Bacterial Colonization and Persistence

The oral microbiome in humans is distinctly different from that of other species. Similarly, the human oral microbiome is distinctly different from that of other body compartments, such as the skin, intestine, and vagina [48]. The oral microbiome comprises a highly diverse microbial population, involving more than 700 species [49]. Furthermore, within the oral microbiome, the dental biofilm has its own microbiome characterized by strong tooth surface adhering streptococci and Actinomyces [50]. Adhesion is essential for colonisation within the oral cavity, and it is regulated primarily by the host and host receptors on the mucosal surface and teeth. In fact, the host selectively, very early after birth, allows the microorganisms that best fit to the receptors of each individual and the specific environment of the oral cavity to colonize. The receptor interaction is mediated by microbial adhesins, which are surface structures such as fimbriae, capsule, lipopolysaccharides and others.

In the area of the gingival crevice, the microenvironment is different from other parts of the tooth surface, with the major nutrition probably coming from gingival crevicular fluid (GCF). Since GCF, in contrast to saliva, does not contain any sugars, the main source of nutrition for the microbiota in this niche are the proteins. Hence, the main metabolic pathway is proteolytic, thus favouring the proteolytic rather than the saccharolytic microorganisms. In addition, the GCF, which is a serum exudate, also contains a number of growth supporting factors such as vitamins (e.g., K-vitamin or menadione), hormones (e.g., oestrogen) and specific serum proteins/peptides (e.g., hemin) all favouring many of the fastidious Gram-negative anaerobes that adapt and grow concomitantly with gingival inflammation and deepening gingival pockets [24,50,51].

Gingival inflammation typically results in a deepening of the gingival pocket owing to swelling, oedema and resulting in increased flow of GCF. This has an impact on the type of colonizing and growing bacteria since it further provides nutritious advantages to proteolytic species. Furthermore, the lowering redox potential (Eh), which is arising from the swelling, favours the anaerobes. In contrast to the supragingival plaque, the adhesion of the microorganisms does not play a crucial role in the gingival pocket and motile bacteria (*Treponema, Campylobacter, Selenomonas* spp.) are able to establish themselves by mechanical retention [50]. The GCF contains humoral defence factors (antibodies, complement, antimicrobial peptides) as well as inflammatory cells such as neutrophils and monocytes. This selects for bacteria that can escape phagocytosis and killing by producing anti-phagocytic capsules (*P. gingivalis*) or leukotoxins (*A. actinomycetemcomitans*), or that simply are proteolytic enough to degrade most proteins, including humoral antimicrobial factors such as immunoglobulins (IgG), complement factors, or antimicrobial host defence peptides [52]. The exudate also contains lysozyme, an enzyme directed towards the peptidoglycan of the bacterial cell wall, which is protected by the outer membrane of Gram-negative microorganisms (Gram-positives lack such outer membrane). Consequently, Gram-negatives appear to have a higher survival rate in the inflamed gingival pocket. Inevitably, inflamed gingival pockets contain a microbiota dominated by Gram-negative, anaerobic, proteolytic, and motile bacteria as they are favoured by and adapted to the changing pocket environment (Table 1). This character of the subgingival plaque microbiota has been repeatedly shown in numerous studies for decades using microscopic-, culture- and molecular biology methods [8,53–56]. The composition of the subgingival microbiota can thus convincingly be explained as a result of a changing ecology involving only commensals (essentially non-pathogenic microorganisms) that are adapting to the new environment [8].

6. Factors Promoting Gingival Inflammation

6.1. Bacterial Metabolites as Pro-Inflammatory and/or Cytotoxic Agents

The products of bacterial metabolic processes, the metabolites, can be used by the bacteria for the construction of new macromolecules, but may also remain by-products with cytotoxic potential and take part in the host-microbe interplay. In a combined metagenome/metatranscriptome analysis that compared active and non-progressing sites in periodontitis patients it was confirmed that proteolysis is associated with progressing periodontal sites [57]. Such bacterial metabolism results in the formation of various compounds, some of which are suggested to participate in the pathogenesis of periodontitis [58].

Bacterial hydrogen sulfide (H_2S) is formed predominantly by degradation of the amino acid L-cysteine or the peptide glutathione by various bacterial species that are associated with periodontitis [59]. H_2S is also formed from sulfate by sulfate reducing bacteria. It is a volatile sulfur compound that has been shown to induce the secretion of the pro-inflammatory cytokines IL-1β and IL-18 in monocytes in vitro through the formation of the NLRP3 inflammasome (Figure 1) [59]. These and other pro-inflammatory cytokines are necessary to sustain or even strengthen the inflammatory reactions in the gingiva. Furthermore, H_2S can induce apoptosis in human gingival fibroblasts [60] and split disulfide bonds in host proteins. These mechanisms, that in different ways trigger inflammatory reactions, are proposed to contribute to the disruption of homeostasis between host cells and bacteria, and to participate in the development of disease. In support of this notion, the sulfur compound metabolic processes have been shown to be enhanced in periodontitis progressing sites [57]. Other volatile sulfur compounds, such as methyl mercaptan, dimethyl disulfide, and dimethyl sulfide, are formed from the degradation of L-methionine among other metabolic pathways, and have similarly been suggested to participate in the host-microbiome crosstalk during the induction and progression of periodontal disease [61].

Additional products of the catabolism of L-cysteine and L-methionine are, together with H_2S and methyl mercaptan, ammonia and pyruvate. Ammonia (NH_3), a product of numerous metabolic processes that take place in the periodontal pocket including the transformation of arginine or lysine [62], is suggested to, apart from its effects on pH, also affect neutrophil function [63]. Apart from ammonia, the degradation of arginine can also, result in the by-product and amino acid citrulline [62]. Pyruvate can be degraded into acetic acid or formic acid for energy production [64].

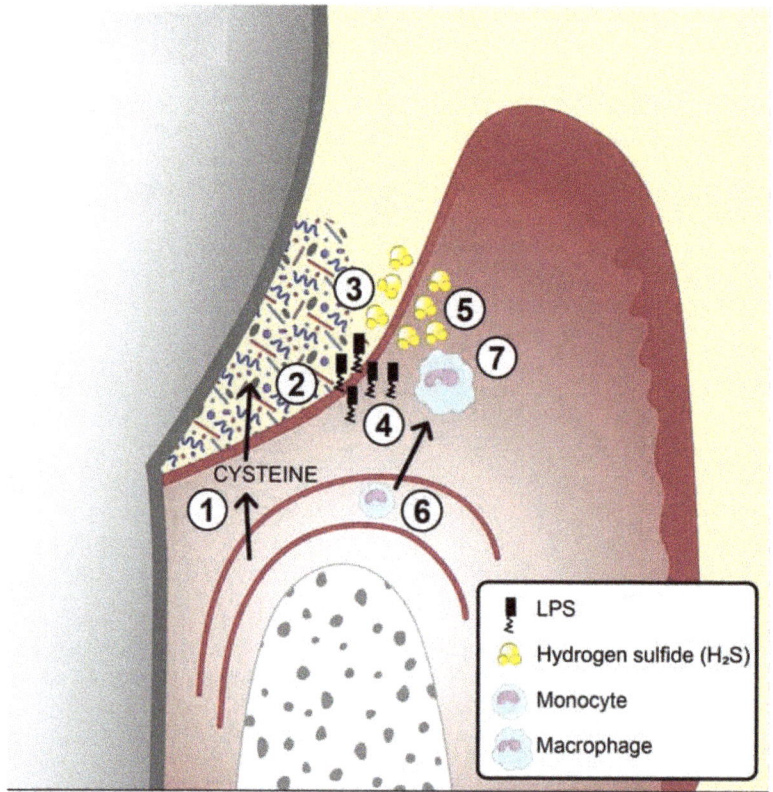

Figure 1. A schematic figure of an inflamed gingival pocket with subgingival plaque (biofilm) and the two signals that lead to the production and secretion of IL-1ß and IL-18 from monocytes/macrophages as reprinted from Basic et al. [59]. The numbers in the figure indicates the following: 1. Serum exudate from blood vessels containing serum proteins, peptides and amino acids including cysteine. 2. The exudate (gingival crevicular fluid, GCF) continues through the thin pocket epithelium (junctional epithelium) into the subgingival pocket. 3. The subgingival plaque, containing numerous, mainly Gram-negative, anaerobic bacteria with proteolytic capacity, degrade proteins, peptides and amino acids including cysteine. 4. Growing Gram-negative anaerobes release lipopolysaccharides (LPS) that penetrate the junctional epithelium into gingival connective tissues. 5. Growing Gram-negative anaerobes (*Fusobacterium* spp. *P. gingivalis*, *Treponema* spp., and others) produce metabolites e.g., hydrogen sulfide (H_2S). 6. The inflammatory lesion attracts monocytes that migrate into the connective tissue and differentiate to macrophages. 7. The effect of LPS and H_2S on macrophages and the subsequent production of the pro-inflammatory cytokines IL-1β and IL-18.

Various carboxylic acids, i.e., acetic acid, butyric acid, formic acid, isobutyric acid, isovaleric acid, lactic acid, propionic acid, phenylacetic acid, succinic acid, and valeric acid are by-products of the deamination of amino acids to generate energy. The presence of many of these have been found to be elevated at inflamed and diseased periodontal sites [65–68]. Comparably to other metabolites, also these mainly short-chain fatty acids have been suggested to act as potent and modifying factors in periodontitis. Butyric acid (Table 1) has for instance been shown to be capable of inducing apoptosis and autophagic cell death in gingival epithelial cells [69], to induce apoptosis in inflamed fibroblasts [70], to induce ROS production, and to impair the cell growth of gingival fibroblasts [71]. These effects stimulate inflammation and are thus, thought to contribute to initiation and the prolongation of periodontitis [66]. Interestingly, many of these metabolites are recognized by specific free fatty acid receptors (FFAR) on leukocytes such as neutrophils and potently attract and activate these cells [72]. This receptor group all bind short-chain fatty acids and include FFA1R (earlier known as GPR40), FFA2R (earlier known as GPR43) and FFA3R (earlier known as GPR41). Such recognition of free fatty acids likely influences both metabolic and immunologic processes [73], and although there has been quite some interest on how free fatty acids produced by the gut microbiota affect health and disease [74], to our knowledge, nothing is known regarding oral bacteria and whether free fatty acid production has bearing on inflammatory reactions in the gingiva.

Apart from the formation of new macromolecules and the interplay with the host, the metabolites also contribute to environmental changes that provide the transformations that are needed for the bacterial shift from homeostasis. Sulfur compounds are, for instance, reducing agents that contribute to lowering the redox potential which favor obligately anaerobic bacteria. Similarly, ammonia is an advocated contributor to the slightly alkaline pH of the periodontal pocket. Other metabolites that have been discussed in the literature as bacterial cytotoxic end-products playing a mediating role in periodontal disease pathogenesis include indole, amines (derivatives of ammonia), and the polyamine cadaverine, which is produced from lysine and shown to be elevated at diseased sites [75].

6.2. Bacterial Cell-Wall Constituents as Pro-inflammatory Factors

Bacterial cell-wall constituents such as short and long fimbriae, outer membrane vesicles and endotoxin (lipopolysaccharide; LPS) have been proposed in various ways to interact with (or even to cause subversion of) the inflammatory response [76,77]. Most attention for immune modulation has been directed toward LPS that builds up the outer membrane of all Gram-negative bacteria and consists of a Lipid A moiety, a core polysaccharide, and a polysaccharide chain of repeating sugar subunits. The latter is an important antigen (O-antigen) that has been used for classification of several enteric genera. LPS is a very immunoreactive molecule and seen as a molecular pattern recognized by potential host organisms—genome-encoded receptors capable of reacting to LPS are found in organisms ranging from plants to mammals [78]. In humans, LPS is sensed primarily by toll-like receptor (TLR) 4, which is expressed by immune cells, but also by a wide variety of other cell types. When bound by LPS, TLR4 activates the pro-inflammatory transcription factor NF-κB that enters the nucleus and initiates gene transcription (Figure 2).

This is a pivotal event that regulates the production of multiple pro-inflammatory cytokines [78]. The broad pro-inflammatory response triggered by NF-κB makes LPS a primary candidate for immune-modulation of gingival inflammation. Since all Gram-negative bacteria release LPS, they may all be involved in triggering/sustaining periodontal inflammation. However, the potency of LPS to trigger inflammation varies among different bacteria, and although this has been studied extensively for *P. gingivalis* [79], less is known about the bioactivity of LPS from other Gram-negatives residing in inflamed gingival pockets.

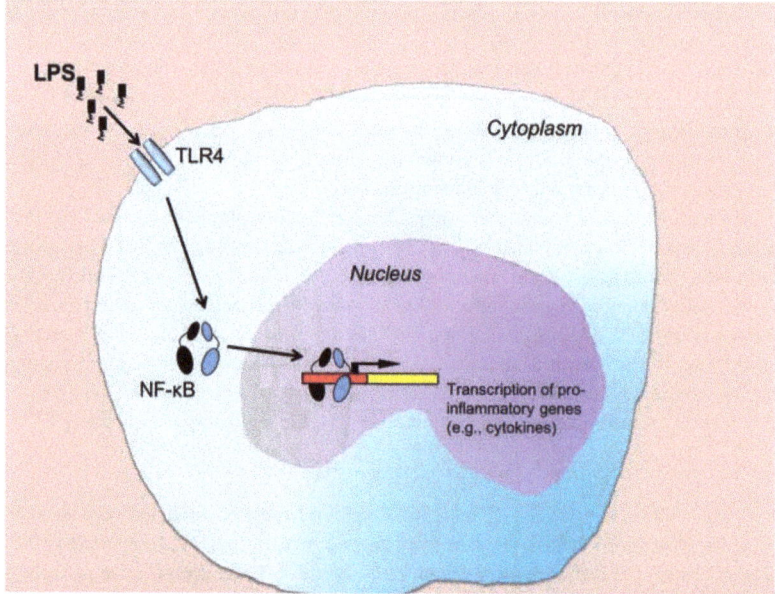

Figure 2. LPS from Gram-negative bacteria bind and activate TLR4 which leads to the activation and translocation from the cytoplasm of the transcription factor NF-κB. Inside the nucleus, NF-κB initiates the transcription of a wide variety of pro-inflammatory genes, e.g., those encoding for pro-inflammatory cytokines.

7. Invasion and Factors that Promote Tissue Degradation

As mentioned above, bacterial invasion is a key process in order to define infections by commensal bacteria, and although invasion seems well established for, e.g., peri-implantitis, it is less clear if it occurs and if it is of importance for chronic periodontitis. How bacteria penetrate through the epithelium and reach the gingival connective tissues is also unclear [80,81], but the pathways commonly discussed [81,82] are: the intercellular route, the intracellular route and by trauma.

7.1. The Intercellular Route

An intercellular route is suggested to take place primarily by motile species, e.g., spirochetes [82]. The junctional epithelium is non-keratinized and thin (4–5 cells thick), and in a state of inflammation, the cells are not tightly joined in order to facilitate gingival exudate and migration of neutrophils and monocytes through the gingival barrier. It is hypothesized that this intercellular passage also allows motile bacteria such as *Treponema* and *Campylobacter* species to penetrate the barrier. *Treponema* spp. and *P. gingivalis* produce specific gingipains that can degrade epithelial junctional proteins (E-cadherin and occludin), and this impairs the junction-related structures [83,84].

Invasion is more likely to take place if the epithelial barrier (junctional epithelium) is disrupted in the case of ulceration. In acute necrotizing ulcerative gingivitis (ANUG) spirochetes are shown to invade the underlying connective tissue by motility [85]. A similar situation is also seen in peri-implantitis where the epithelium fails to cover the connective tissues of the apical part of the peri-implant pocket [46,86]. The periodontal abscess is another example of invasion into the tissues by bacterial growth, and the abscess can sometimes even lead to fistula formation. Invasion in these examples is due to bacterial multiplication and expansion, and it is associated with heavy neutrophil attraction and suppuration, and sometimes symptoms characteristic of an acute infection.

7.2. The Intracellular Route

The intracellular route has gained more attention since it was noticed that viable and non-keratinized epithelial cells contain bacteria. Buccal epithelial cells regularly contain bacterial cells, mainly streptococci [87]. Interestingly, *P. gingivalis* and other periodontal bacteria have also been shown in such cells [88]. *T. forsythia, Prevotella intermedia* and *C. rectus* have been identified inside crevicular epithelial cells in vivo [89], and this uptake is mediated by receptor interaction between the bacteria and the epithelial cells [90]. Fimbriae (long and short fimbriae) is suggested to play a crucial role in bacterial invasion of cells and periodontal tissues through receptor interaction between the fimbriae and host cells [76]. *P. gingivalis* long fimbriae can be divided based on the *fimA* gene into 6 different subtypes of which *fimA* II and IV were more prevalent in periodontitis while *fimA* type I is more prevalent in healthy periodontal tissues [91]. Fimbriated *P. gingivalis* have been shown to be more efficient than fimbriae-deficient *P. gingivalis* to enter human dendritic cells in vitro [92], while Type II fimbriae were associated with increased proinflammatory and invasive activities in macrophages [76]. Interestingly, in one study a Type-1 fimbriae *P. gingivalis* strain induced more bone loss than a Type-II *P. gingivalis* strain in a mouse model [93]. Nevertheless, the importance of fimbriae for tissue invasion in the complex interaction between the subgingival microbiota and the host response in humans remains to be elucidated.

7.3. Invasion by Trauma

Bacterial invasion of the pocket epithelium and the underlying connective tissue in gingival biopsies from patients with periodontitis has been reported using various methods [81]. These studies clearly show presence of various periodontitis associated bacteria intracellularly in epithelial cells as well as in the connective tissue, but without explaining whether they have passed the barrier actively or accidentally by trauma (e.g., while taking the biopsies). Bacteria are commonly pushed into the connective tissues during manipulations and hygienic procedures (tooth brushing, flossing, tooth picks) and chewing. Dental hygienists or dentists, during cleaning and treatment procedures (depuration, scaling, ultrasonication, probing, periodontal surgery and tooth extractions), frequently cause the spread of microorganisms into the blood stream. Bacteremia during dental procedures is thus a well-known phenomenon, and poor oral hygiene, with an abundance of plaque and inflammation, increases the likelihood of bacterial spread out in the tissues. It is likely that most people have bacteremia daily without any (severe) consequences but it is also possible that bacteria can survive within the periodontal tissues and not being immediately eliminated by the host defense.

7.4. Tissue Degrading Factors

Tissue degrading or histolytic enzymes produced by bacteria were previously thought to be directly responsible for periodontal tissue breakdown [94], comparably to similar enzymes of pathogenic tissue invading bacteria such as *Clostridium histolyticum, Staphylococcus aureus* and *Streptococcus pyogenes* (Group A streptococci) [94]. Hyaluronidase ("spreading factor"), chondroitin sulphatase, and beta-glucuronidase produced by various oral bacteria such as streptococci, peptostreptococci, and corynebacteria (diphteroids) were thought to facilitate the spread of infections by degrading tissue components. Similarly, various bacterial proteases including collagenases were thought to play a major role by degrading tissue constituents in infections involving anaerobic proteolytic bacteria [94]. It was tempting to argue that collagenases and gingipains (previously termed "trypsin-like") produced by several *Porphyromonas* species (e.g., *P. gingivalis* and *P. gulae*) degrading almost any protein in vitro also had a role in periodontal pathology. Although, realizing that host defense cells, e.g., neutrophils and macrophages, also produce similar enzymes, the possibility that bacterial enzymes contribute to tissue degradation has been diminished.

8. Factors for Evasion of Host Defence

The host reacts extensively to the microbial challenge by employing the inflammatory reaction and assembling defense factors such as neutrophils, complement factors, and antibodies in the exudate and gingival pocket [95]. Microorganisms with the capacity to evade such host factors will increase their survival rate. As mentioned above, proteolytic enzymes may split or degrade the host's defense molecules such as immunoglobulins and complement [96], but there are also more sophisticated mechanisms for the evasion of host defense.

8.1. Exotoxins

Toxins that destroy leukocytes, leukotoxins, are well-known virulence factors found in several pathogenic bacteria such as the PV-leucocidin in *Staphylococcus aureus* [97] and *Fusobacterium necrophorum* [98]. This explains the invasive and abscess-promoting character of these pathogens. Therefore, the leukotoxin-producing microorganism, *A. actinomycetemcomitans*, among the periodontal bacteria, has been extensively studied due to this particular factor [99,100]. The importance of leukotoxin in *A. actinomycetemcomitans* was emphasized when discovering the high toxic JP2 clone, which produces highly elevated levels of leukotoxin. Interestingly, Höglund et al. [101] correctly predicted that children of a Ghanaian cohort harboring *A. actinomycetemcomitans* and the high-toxic clone (JP2) in particular, at periodontal sites, had significantly more periodontal breakdown after 2 years compared with baseline, indicating a specific impact of the JP2 clone on the disease progression. The leukotoxin explains the specific ability of this bacterium to survive or escape the host's defense (neutrophils present in the gingival pockets), but it does not explain the periodontal breakdown that is associated with this bacterium in aggressive forms of periodontitis in children and adolescents [102]. The fact that the toxin is both membrane-associated and secreted may be important since (at least) the secreted form would likely create a local niche free from viable neutrophils, which would benefit all bacteria present at this site.

8.2. Capsule Formation

The formation of an anti-phagocytic capsule is a well-known virulence strategy of many pathogenic microorganisms. *Streptococcus pneumoniae* and *Haemophilus influence* are exclusively dependent on capsule formation and vaccination of children towards their capsular antigens is today a reality [103,104]. Capsules are produced by many Gram-negative anaerobic rods, e.g., *Bacteroides, Prevotella,* and *Porphyromonas* [105,106]. The capsule is produced to escape phagocytosis and thereby intracellular killing by neutrophils and macrophages. The inability of the host's defense to kill capsulated bacteria may result in spread of infections and to complications such as sepsis [107]. Six capsular serotypes have been identified among periodontal *P. gingivalis* isolates (Table 1). Two capsular types, K1 and K6, seem to include isolates with a lower adhesion capacity to human leukocytes in vitro than the other capsular types [105,108]. However, in vivo evidence supporting that any of the capsular types would be more associated with periodontitis than others are lacking.

9. Systemic Implications of Periodontal Bacteria

Bacteraemia and focal infections from the oral cavity have been associated with teeth and oral conditions for more than hundred years [109]. Formerly, the total extraction of all teeth was a common way to avoid future problems and full dentures was the only option for adults, and still is in many countries in the world. Incomplete endodontic treatment was thought to be the major cause of focal infections and apical periodontitis is still a suspected (by the medical profession) major point of entry for oral bacteria into the blood stream and further to various organs of the body. Today, the systemic effects from marginal periodontitis is considered to be much more important [109]. Not only bacteria as such but also products from subgingival bacteria (e.g., metabolites and endotoxins), and inflammatory mediators produced locally in the periodontal tissues, are being linked to the chronic inflammation seen in a number of systemic diseases such as atherosclerosis, diabetes, preterm birth, rheumatoid arthritis and Alzheimer's disease [5,110]. Especially, the association between periodontitis and putative periodontal pathogens to Alzheimer's disease has been in focus during the last decade and *P. gingivalis* LPS and outer-membrane vesicles have been suggested to be accumulated in brain tissues of patients with Alzheimer's disease [77,111]. Most studies linking periodontitis to systemic diseases are association studies and it is less clear what (if any) unique contribution periodontitis might have that would not be found for other chronic inflammatory diseases in the body (e.g., in the gut).

However, one disease where the connection to periodontitis appears more solid than a mere association between the two diseases, is rheumatoid arthritis (RA), a widespread systemic inflammatory disease that is mainly manifested as peripheral polyarthritis (i.e., inflammation of peripheral joints) and that affects up to 1% of the global population [112]. RA is a heterogeneous disease but the majority of cases feature auto-antibodies directed towards citrullinated epitopes, so-called anti-citrullinated protein antibodies (ACPAs). Citrullination is a biochemical post-translational modification where arginine residues of peptides and proteins are converted into citrulline residues. In general, protein citrullination is of great physiological importance and endogenous citrullination is ascertained by a family of human enzymes known as peptidylarginine deiminases (PADs), some of which are primarily located immune cells, such as neutrophils. PAD-mediated citrullination of arginine residues may create neo-epitopes that could give rise to the development of ACPAs and one major research questions in RA deal with how, when, and where tolerance is broken to allow for the generation of ACPAs.

A. acinomycetemcomitans has been shown to trigger dysregulated citrullination of proteins, a process mediated by the activation and release of endogenous neutrophil PAD by the actions of the bacterial leukotoxin [113]. Although the pore-forming leukotoxin of *A. actinomycetemcomitans* is exclusive among oral bacteria, pore formation is by no means a unique feature of bacterial toxins in general. Additionally, *P. gingivalis* has been implicated as a potentially even more interesting link between periodontitis and RA when it was found that it expresses a bacterial PAD, typically referred to as PPAD, to distinguish it from the human isoforms [114]. PPAD seems to be rather uniquely expressed by *P. gingivalis* among the bacteria that interact with humans and it has the ability to create citrullinated neo-epitopes that are recognized by ACPAs from RA patients. Interestingly, *P. gingivalis* appears especially fit to do this, since the PPAD is specific for C-terminal arginine residues and such peptides are typically generated by the gingipains. Thus, these two *P. gingivalis* enzymes (PPAD and gingipains) appear to work in concert, in a way that maximize the levels of citrullinated epitopes which might thereby break tolerance and facilitate the generation of ACPAs [112].

10. Conclusions

Inflammation in the gingiva (gingivitis) is a normal host tissue response (a physiological inflammation) triggered by ordinary commensal microorganisms and the products (metabolites, endotoxins) released from them during growth. Periodontitis is a pathological inflammatory disease, as a response to years of prolonged exposure to a polymicrobial community in the gingival/periodontal pocket, involving tissue responses with alternating destructive (damage) and healing (repair) phases, but with a net loss of attachment and bone. The infectious nature of the microbes, and to what extent specific bacterial species, with specific virulence factors capable of interference with host defense and tissue repair, play in disease onset and progression, are still unclear. Most of the factors that used to be discussed in terms of virulence (proteases, LPS, invasive ability, fimbriae, capsule, leukotoxin) among microorganisms commonly associated with periodontitis should rather be termed survival factors, since they do not necessarily constitute factors for pathogenicity and damage but for the living, growth, and survival of the bacteria in deep, inflamed periodontal pockets. One exception is the leukotoxin produced by *A. actinomycetemcomitans* (and the JP2 genotype where clinical evidence support a causative role in disease progression) [101] and although the mechanism whereby the leukotoxin leads to tissue damage is still not known, this bacterial species best fulfils the designation of a putative periodontal pathogen in the human oral microbiota.

Author Contributions: G.D., A.B. and J.B. reviewed the literature and wrote the review.

Funding: No funding was raised for preparing this review.

Acknowledgments: (Figure 1 is published in an Open Access journal and is distributed under the terms of the Creative Commons Attribution ver. 4.0 International License https://creativecommons.org/licenses/by/4.0/, which is hereby acknowledged.

Conflicts of Interest: The authors report no conflicts of interest.

References

1. Hashim, D.; Cionca, N.; Combescure, C.; Mombelli, A. The diagnosis of peri-implantitis: A systematic review on the predictive value of bleeding on probing. *Clin. Oral Implants Res.* **2018**, *29* (Suppl. S16), 276–293. [CrossRef]
2. Teles, R.; Teles, F.; Frias-Lopez, J.; Paster, B.; Haffajee, A. Lessons learned and unlearned in periodontal microbiology. *Periodontology 2000* **2013**, *62*, 95–162. [CrossRef] [PubMed]
3. Baelum, V.; Lopez, R. Periodontal disease epidemiology—Learned and unlearned? *Periodontology 2000* **2013**, *62*, 37–58. [CrossRef] [PubMed]
4. Kinane, D.F.; Stathopoulou, P.G.; Papapanou, P.N. Periodontal diseases. *Nat. Rev. Dis. Primers* **2017**, *3*, 17038. [CrossRef]
5. Bui, F.Q.; Almeida-da-Silva, C.L.C.; Huynh, B.; Trinh, A.; Liu, J.; Woodward, J.; Asadi, H.; Ojcius, D.M. Association between periodontal pathogens and systemic disease. *Biomed. J.* **2019**, *42*, 27–35. [CrossRef] [PubMed]
6. Loe, H.; Theilade, E.; Jensen, S.B. Experimental gingivitis in man. *J. Periodontal.* **1965**, *36*, 177–187. [CrossRef] [PubMed]
7. Socransky, S.S.; Haffajee, A.D. Evidence of bacterial etiology: A historical perspective. *Periodontology 2000* **1994**, *5*, 7–25. [CrossRef] [PubMed]
8. Socransky, S.S.; Haffajee, A.D. Periodontal microbial ecology. *Periodontology 2000* **2005**, *38*, 135–187. [CrossRef] [PubMed]
9. Socransky, S.S. Criteria for the infectious agents in dental caries and periodontal disease. *J. Clin. Periodontal.* **1979**, *6*, 16–21. [CrossRef] [PubMed]
10. Loesche, W.J. The therapeutic use of antimicrobial agents in patients with periodontal disease. *Scand. J. Infect. Dis. Suppl.* **1985**, *46*, 106–114. [PubMed]
11. Page, R.C.; Kornman, K.S. The pathogenesis of human periodontitis: An introduction. *Periodontology 2000* **1997**, *14*, 9–11. [CrossRef] [PubMed]
12. Meyle, J.; Chapple, I. Molecular aspects of the pathogenesis of periodontitis. *Periodontology 2000* **2015**, *69*, 7–17. [CrossRef] [PubMed]
13. Haber, J.; Wattles, J.; Crowley, M.; Mandell, R.; Joshipura, K.; Kent, R.L. Evidence for cigarette smoking as a major risk factor for periodontitis. *J. Periodontal.* **1993**, *64*, 16–23. [CrossRef] [PubMed]
14. Emrich, L.J.; Shlossman, M.; Genco, R.J. Periodontal disease in non-insulin-dependent diabetes mellitus. *J. Periodontal.* **1991**, *62*, 123–131. [CrossRef] [PubMed]
15. Loos, B.G.; Papantonopoulos, G.; Jepsen, S.; Laine, M.L. What is the contribution of genetics to periodontal risk? *Dent. Clin.* **2015**, *59*, 761–780. [CrossRef]
16. Nibali, L.; Bayliss-Chapman, J.; Almofareh, S.A.; Zhou, Y.; Divaris, K.; Vieira, A.R. What Is the heritability of periodontitis? A systematic review. *J. Dent. Res.* **2019**, *98*, 632–641. [CrossRef]
17. Kassebaum, N.J.; Bernabe, E.; Dahiya, M.; Bhandari, B.; Murray, C.J.; Marcenes, W. Global burden of severe periodontitis in 1990–2010: A systematic review and meta-regression. *J. Dent. Res.* **2014**, *93*, 1045–1053. [CrossRef]
18. Larsson, L. Current concepts of epigenetics and its role in periodontitis. *Curr. Oral Health Rep.* **2017**, *4*, 286–293. [CrossRef]
19. Luo, Y.; Peng, X.; Duan, D.; Liu, C.; Xu, X.; Zhou, X. Epigenetic regulations in the pathogenesis of periodontitis. *Curr. Stem Cell Res. Ther.* **2018**, *13*, 144–150. [CrossRef]
20. De-La-Torre, J.; Quindos, G.; Marcos-Arias, C.; Marichalar-Mendia, X.; Gainza, M.L.; Eraso, E.; Acha-Sagredo, A.; Aguirre-Urizar, J.M. Oral Candida colonization in patients with chronic periodontitis. Is there any relationship? *Rev. Iberoam. Micol.* **2018**, *35*, 134–139. [CrossRef]

21. Slots, J. Periodontitis: Facts, fallacies and the future. *Periodontology 2000* **2017**, *75*, 7–23. [CrossRef] [PubMed]
22. Rosier, B.T.; Marsh, P.D.; Mira, A. Resilience of the oral microbiota in health: Mechanisms that prevent dysbiosis. *J. Dent. Res.* **2018**, *97*, 371–380. [CrossRef] [PubMed]
23. Lamont, R.J.; Koo, H.; Hajishengallis, G. The oral microbiota: Dynamic communities and host interactions. *Nat. Rev. Microbiol.* **2018**, *16*, 745–759. [CrossRef] [PubMed]
24. Kilian, M.; Chapple, I.L.; Hannig, M.; Marsh, P.D.; Meuric, V.; Pedersen, A.M.; Tonetti, M.S.; Wade, W.G.; Zaura, E. The oral microbiome—An update for oral healthcare professionals. *Br. Dent. J.* **2016**, *221*, 657–666. [CrossRef] [PubMed]
25. Lopez, R.; Hujoel, P.; Belibasakis, G.N. On putative periodontal pathogens: An epidemiological perspective. *Virulence* **2015**, *6*, 249–257. [CrossRef] [PubMed]
26. Dahlen, G.; Manji, F.; Baelum, V.; Fejerskov, O. Putative periodontopathogens in "diseased" and "non-diseased" persons exhibiting poor oral hygiene. *J. Clin. Periodontal.* **1992**, *19*, 35–42. [CrossRef]
27. Socransky, S.S.; Haffajee, A.D.; Cugini, M.A.; Smith, C.; Kent, R.L., Jr. Microbial complexes in subgingival plaque. *J. Clin. Periodontal.* **1998**, *25*, 134–144. [CrossRef]
28. Lamont, R.J.; Jenkinson, H.F. Life below the gum line: Pathogenic mechanisms of *Porphyromonas gingivalis*. *Microbiol. Mol. Biol. Rev.* **1998**, *62*, 1244–1263.
29. Holt, S.C.; Ebersole, J.L. Porphyromonas gingivalis, *Treponema denticola*, and *Tannerella forsythia*: The "red complex", a prototype polybacterial pathogenic consortium in periodontitis. *Periodontology 2000* **2005**, *38*, 72–122. [CrossRef]
30. Fine, D.H.; Patil, A.G.; Velusamy, S.K. *Aggregatibacter actinomycetemcomitans* (Aa) under the radar: Myths and misunderstandings of Aa and its role in aggressive periodontitis. *Front. Immunol.* **2019**, *10*, 728. [CrossRef]
31. Listgarten, M.A.; Hellden, L. Relative distribution of bacteria at clinically healthy and periodontally diseased sites in humans. *J. Clin. Periodontal.* **1978**, *5*, 115–132. [CrossRef] [PubMed]
32. Huo, Y.B.; Chan, Y.; Lacap-Bugler, D.C.; Mo, S.; Woo, P.C.Y.; Leung, W.K.; Watt, R.M. Multilocus sequence analysis of phylogroup 1 and 2 oral treponeme strains. *Appl. Environ. Microbiol.* **2017**, *83*, e02499-16. [CrossRef] [PubMed]
33. You, M.; Mo, S.; Leung, W.K.; Watt, R.M. Comparative analysis of oral treponemes associated with periodontal health and disease. *BMC Infect. Dis.* **2013**, *13*, 174. [CrossRef] [PubMed]
34. Haubek, D.; Ennibi, O.K.; Poulsen, K.; Vaeth, M.; Poulsen, S.; Kilian, M. Risk of aggressive periodontitis in adolescent carriers of the JP2 clone of *Aggregatibacter* (*Actinobacillus*) *actinomycetemcomitans* in Morocco: A prospective longitudinal cohort study. *Lancet* **2008**, *371*, 237–242. [CrossRef]
35. Perez-Chaparro, P.J.; Goncalves, C.; Figueiredo, L.C.; Faveri, M.; Lobao, E.; Tamashiro, N.; Duarte, P.; Feres, M. Newly identified pathogens associated with periodontitis: A systematic review. *J. Dent. Res.* **2014**, *93*, 846–858. [CrossRef] [PubMed]
36. Wade, W.G. Has the use of molecular methods for the characterization of the human oral microbiome changed our understanding of the role of bacteria in the pathogenesis of periodontal disease? *J. Clin. Periodontal.* **2011**, *38* (Suppl. S11), 7–16. [CrossRef] [PubMed]
37. Curtis, M.A. Periodontal microbiology—The lid's off the box again. *J. Dent. Res.* **2014**, *93*, 840–842. [CrossRef]
38. Charalampakis, G.; Dahlen, G.; Carlen, A.; Leonhardt, A. Bacterial markers vs. clinical markers to predict progression of chronic periodontitis: A 2-yr prospective observational study. *Eur. J. Oral Sci.* **2013**, *121*, 394–402. [CrossRef]
39. Casadevall, A.; Pirofski, L.A. Virulence factors and their mechanisms of action: The view from a damage-response framework. *J. Water Health* **2009**, *7* (Suppl. S1), S2–S18. [CrossRef]
40. Isenberg, H.D. Pathogenicity and virulence: Another view. *Clin. Microbiol. Rev.* **1988**, *1*, 40–53. [CrossRef]
41. Anonymous. *Dorland's Medical Dictionary*; Saunders: Philadelphia, PA, USA, 2007.
42. Manji, F.; Dahlen, G.; Fejerskov, O. Caries and periodontitis: Contesting the conventional wisdom on their aetiology. *Caries Res.* **2018**, *52*, 548–564. [CrossRef] [PubMed]
43. Dahlen, G. Microbiology and treatment of dental abscesses and periodontal-endodontic lesions. *Periodontology 2000* **2002**, *28*, 206–239. [CrossRef] [PubMed]
44. Lewis, M.A.; MacFarlane, T.W.; McGowan, D.A. Quantitative bacteriology of acute dento-alveolar abscesses. *J. Med. Microbiol.* **1986**, *21*, 101–104. [CrossRef] [PubMed]
45. Charalampakis, G.; Belibasakis, G.N. Microbiome of peri-implant infections: Lessons from conventional, molecular and metagenomic analyses. *Virulence* **2015**, *6*, 183–187. [CrossRef] [PubMed]

46. Berglundh, T.; Gislason, O.; Lekholm, U.; Sennerby, L.; Lindhe, J. Histopathological observations of human periimplantitis lesions. *J. Clin. Periodontal.* **2004**, *31*, 341–347. [CrossRef] [PubMed]
47. Dahlen, G.; Fabricius, L.; Holm, S.E.; Moller, A. Interactions within a collection of eight bacterial strains isolated from a monkey dental root canal. *Oral Microbiol. Immunol.* **1987**, *2*, 164–170. [CrossRef] [PubMed]
48. Project, C.H.M. Structure, function and diversity of the healthy human microbiome. *Nature* **2012**, *486*, 207–214. [CrossRef]
49. Verma, D.; Garg, P.K.; Dubey, A.K. Insights into the human oral microbiome. *Arch. Microbiol.* **2018**, *200*, 525–540. [CrossRef] [PubMed]
50. Marsh, P.; Lewis, M.; Williams, D.; Marsh, P.; Martin, M.; Lewis, M.; Williams, D. *Oral Microbiology*, 5th ed.; Churchill Livingstone: Edinburgh, UK, 2009.
51. Carlsson, J. Growth and nutrition as ecological factors. In *Oral Bacterial Ecology. The Molecular Basis*; Kuramitsu, H.K., Ellen, R.P., Eds.; Horizon Scientific Press: Norfolk, UK, 2000; pp. 68–130.
52. Devine, D.A.; Cosseau, C. Host defense peptides in the oral cavity. *Adv. Appl. Microbiol.* **2008**, *63*, 281–322. [CrossRef] [PubMed]
53. Theilade, E.; Wright, W.H.; Jensen, S.B.; Loe, H. Experimental gingivitis in man. II. A longitudinal clinical and bacteriological investigation. *J. Periodontal Res.* **1966**, *1*, 1–13. [CrossRef] [PubMed]
54. Moore, L.V.; Moore, W.E.; Cato, E.P.; Smibert, R.M.; Burmeister, J.A.; Best, A.M.; Ranney, R.R. Bacteriology of human gingivitis. *J. Dent. Res.* **1987**, *66*, 989–995. [CrossRef] [PubMed]
55. Slots, J. Subgingival microflora and periodontal disease. *J. Clin. Periodontal.* **1979**, *6*, 351–382. [CrossRef] [PubMed]
56. Griffen, A.L.; Beall, C.J.; Campbell, J.H.; Firestone, N.D.; Kumar, P.S.; Yang, Z.K.; Podar, M.; Leys, E.J. Distinct and complex bacterial profiles in human periodontitis and health revealed by 16S pyrosequencing. *ISME J.* **2012**, *6*, 1176–1185. [CrossRef] [PubMed]
57. Yost, S.; Duran-Pinedo, A.E.; Teles, R.; Krishnan, K.; Frias-Lopez, J. Functional signatures of oral dysbiosis during periodontitis progression revealed by microbial metatranscriptome analysis. *Genome Med.* **2015**, *7*, 27. [CrossRef]
58. Takahashi, N. Oral microbiome metabolism: From "who are they?" to "what are they doing?". *J. Dent. Res.* **2015**, *94*, 1628–1637. [CrossRef]
59. Basic, A.; Alizadehgharib, S.; Dahlen, G.; Dahlgren, U. Hydrogen sulfide exposure induces NLRP3 inflammasome-dependent IL-1beta and IL-18 secretion in human mononuclear leukocytes in vitro. *Clin. Exp. Dent. Res.* **2017**, *3*, 115–120. [CrossRef]
60. Zhang, J.H.; Dong, Z.; Chu, L. Hydrogen sulfide induces apoptosis in human periodontium cells. *J. Periodontal Res.* **2010**, *45*, 71–78. [CrossRef]
61. Nakano, Y.; Yoshimura, M.; Koga, T. Methyl mercaptan production by periodontal bacteria. *Int. Dent. J.* **2002**, *52* (Suppl. S3), 217–220. [CrossRef]
62. Uematsu, H.; Sato, N.; Djais, A.; Hoshino, E. Degradation of arginine by *Slackia exigua* ATCC 700122 and *Cryptobacterium curtum* ATCC 700683. *Oral Microbiol. Immunol.* **2006**, *21*, 381–384. [CrossRef]
63. Niederman, R.; Brunkhorst, B.; Smith, S.; Weinreb, R.N.; Ryder, M.I. Ammonia as a potential mediator of adult human periodontal infection: Inhibition of neutrophil function. *Arch. Oral Biol.* **1990**, *35*, S205–S209. [CrossRef]
64. Uematsu, H.; Sato, N.; Hossain, M.Z.; Ikeda, T.; Hoshino, E. Degradation of arginine and other amino acids by butyrate-producing asaccharolytic anaerobic gram-positive rods in periodontal pockets. *Arch. Oral Biol.* **2003**, *48*, 423–429. [CrossRef]
65. Niederman, R.; Zhang, J.; Kashket, S. Short-chain carboxylic-acid-stimulated, PMN-mediated gingival inflammation. *Crit. Rev. Oral Biol. Med.* **1997**, *8*, 269–290. [CrossRef] [PubMed]
66. Niederman, R.; Buyle-Bodin, Y.; Lu, B.Y.; Robinson, P.; Naleway, C. Short-chain carboxylic acid concentration in human gingival crevicular fluid. *J. Dent. Res.* **1997**, *76*, 575–579. [CrossRef] [PubMed]
67. Qiqiang, L.; Huanxin, M.; Xuejun, G. Longitudinal study of volatile fatty acids in the gingival crevicular fluid of patients with periodontitis before and after nonsurgical therapy. *J. Periodontal Res.* **2012**, *47*, 740–749. [CrossRef] [PubMed]
68. Lu, R.; Meng, H.; Gao, X.; Xu, L.; Feng, X. Effect of non-surgical periodontal treatment on short chain fatty acid levels in gingival crevicular fluid of patients with generalized aggressive periodontitis. *J. Periodontal Res.* **2014**, *49*, 574–583. [CrossRef] [PubMed]

69. Tsuda, H.; Ochiai, K.; Suzuki, N.; Otsuka, K. Butyrate, a bacterial metabolite, induces apoptosis and autophagic cell death in gingival epithelial cells. *J. Periodontal Res.* **2010**, *45*, 626–634. [CrossRef] [PubMed]
70. Kurita-Ochiai, T.; Seto, S.; Suzuki, N.; Yamamoto, M.; Otsuka, K.; Abe, K.; Ochiai, K. Butyric acid induces apoptosis in inflamed fibroblasts. *J. Dent. Res.* **2008**, *87*, 51–55. [CrossRef]
71. Chang, M.C.; Tsai, Y.L.; Chen, Y.W.; Chan, C.P.; Huang, C.F.; Lan, W.C.; Lin, C.C.; Lan, W.H.; Jeng, J.H. Butyrate induces reactive oxygen species production and affects cell cycle progression in human gingival fibroblasts. *J. Periodontal Res.* **2013**, *48*, 66–73. [CrossRef]
72. Bjorkman, L.; Martensson, J.; Winther, M.; Gabl, M.; Holdfeldt, A.; Uhrbom, M.; Bylund, J.; Hojgaard Hansen, A.; Pandey, S.K.; Ulven, T.; et al. The Neutrophil response induced by an agonist for free fatty acid receptor 2 (GPR43) is primed by tumor necrosis factor alpha and by Receptor UNCOUPLING from the cytoskeleton but attenuated by tissue recruitment. *Mol. Cell Biol.* **2016**, *36*, 2583–2595. [CrossRef]
73. Alvarez-Curto, E.; Milligan, G. Metabolism meets immunity: The role of free fatty acid receptors in the immune system. *Biochem. Pharmacol.* **2016**, *114*, 3–13. [CrossRef]
74. Maslowski, K.M.; Vieira, A.T.; Ng, A.; Kranich, J.; Sierro, F.; Yu, D.; Schilter, H.C.; Rolph, M.S.; Mackay, F.; Artis, D.; et al. Regulation of inflammatory responses by gut microbiota and chemoattractant receptor GPR43. *Nature* **2009**, *461*, 1282–1286. [CrossRef] [PubMed]
75. Barnes, V.M.; Teles, R.; Trivedi, H.M.; Devizio, W.; Xu, T.; Mitchell, M.W.; Milburn, M.V.; Guo, L. Acceleration of purine degradation by periodontal diseases. *J. Dent. Res.* **2009**, *88*, 851–855. [CrossRef] [PubMed]
76. Enersen, M.; Nakano, K.; Amano, A. Porphyromonas gingivalis fimbriae. *J. Oral Microbiol.* **2013**, *5*, 20265. [CrossRef] [PubMed]
77. Singhrao, S.K.; Olsen, I. Are *Porphyromonas gingivalis* outer membrane vesicles microbullets for sporadic Alzheimer's disease manifestation? *J. Alzheimers Dis. Rep.* **2018**, *2*, 219–228. [CrossRef] [PubMed]
78. Neyen, C.; Lemaitre, B. Sensing gram-negative bacteria: A phylogenetic perspective. *Curr. Opin. Immunol.* **2016**, *38*, 8–17. [CrossRef] [PubMed]
79. Paramonov, N.; Aduse-Opoku, J.; Hashim, A.; Rangarajan, M.; Curtis, M.A. Identification of the linkage between A-polysaccharide and the core in the A-lipopolysaccharide of *Porphyromonas gingivalis* W50. *J. Bacteriol.* **2015**, *197*, 1735–1746. [CrossRef]
80. Tribble, G.D.; Lamont, R.J. Bacterial invasion of epithelial cells and spreading in periodontal tissue. *Periodontology 2000* **2010**, *52*, 68–83. [CrossRef]
81. Ji, S.; Choi, Y.S.; Choi, Y. Bacterial invasion and persistence: Critical events in the pathogenesis of periodontitis? *J. Periodontal Res.* **2015**, *50*, 570–585. [CrossRef]
82. Lux, R.; Miller, J.N.; Park, N.H.; Shi, W. Motility and chemotaxis in tissue penetration of oral epithelial cell layers by Treponema denticola. *Infect. Immun.* **2001**, *69*, 6276–6283. [CrossRef]
83. Katz, J.; Yang, Q.B.; Zhang, P.; Potempa, J.; Travis, J.; Michalek, S.M.; Balkovetz, D.F. Hydrolysis of epithelial junctional proteins by *Porphyromonas gingivalis* gingipains. *Infect. Immun.* **2002**, *70*, 2512–2518. [CrossRef]
84. Listgarten, M.A. Electron microscopic observations on the bacterial flora of acute necrotizing *Ulcerative gingivitis*. *J. Periodontal.* **1965**, *36*, 328–339. [CrossRef] [PubMed]
85. Listgarten, M.A.; Socransky, S.S. Ultrastructural characteristics of a spirochete in the lesion of acute necrotizing *Ulcerative gingivostomatitis* (Vincent's infection). *Arch. Oral Biol.* **1964**, *9*, 95–96. [CrossRef]
86. Berglundh, T.; Zitzmann, N.U.; Donati, M. Are peri-implantitis lesions different from periodontitis lesions? *J. Clin. Periodontol.* **2011**, *38* (Suppl. S11), 188–202. [CrossRef]
87. Rudney, J.D.; Chen, R.; Zhang, G. Streptococci dominate the diverse flora within buccal cells. *J. Dent. Res.* **2005**, *84*, 1165–1171. [CrossRef] [PubMed]
88. Rudney, J.D.; Chen, R.; Sedgewick, G.J. *Actinobacillus actinomycetemcomitans*, *Porphyromonas gingivalis*, and *Tannerella forsythensis* are components of a polymicrobial intracellular flora within human buccal cells. *J. Dent. Res.* **2005**, *84*, 59–63. [CrossRef] [PubMed]
89. Dibart, S.; Skobe, Z.; Snapp, K.R.; Socransky, S.S.; Smith, C.M.; Kent, R. Identification of bacterial species on or in crevicular epithelial cells from healthy and periodontally diseased patients using DNA-DNA hybridization. *Oral Microbiol. Immunol.* **1998**, *13*, 30–35. [CrossRef] [PubMed]
90. Madianos, P.N.; Papapanou, P.N.; Nannmark, U.; Dahlen, G.; Sandros, J. Porphyromonas gingivalis FDC381 multiplies and persists within human oral epithelial cells in vitro. *Infect. Immun.* **1996**, *64*, 660–664.

91. Amano, A.; Kuboniwa, M.; Nakagawa, I.; Akiyama, S.; Morisaki, I.; Hamada, S. Prevalence of specific genotypes of *Porphyromonas gingivalis* fimA and periodontal health status. *J. Dent. Res.* **2000**, *79*, 1664–1668. [CrossRef]
92. Jotwani, R.; Cutler, C.W. Fimbriated *Porphyromonas gingivalis* is more efficient than fimbria-deficient *P. gingivalis* in entering human dendritic cells in vitro and induces an inflammatory Th1 effector response. *Infect. Immun.* **2004**, *72*, 1725–1732. [CrossRef]
93. Wang, M.; Liang, S.; Hosur, K.B.; Domon, H.; Yoshimura, F.; Amano, A.; Hajishengallis, G. Differential virulence and innate immune interactions of Type I and II fimbrial genotypes of *Porphyromonas gingivalis*. *Oral Microbiol. Immunol.* **2009**, *24*, 478–484. [CrossRef]
94. Burnett, G.W.; Scherp, H.W. *Oral Microbiology and Infectious Disease*, 3rd ed.; The William & Wilkins Company: Baltimore, MD, USA, 1968; p. 982.
95. Attstrom, R.; Schroeder, H.E. Effect of experimental neutropenia on initial gingivitis in dogs. *Scand. J. Dent. Res.* **1979**, *87*, 7–23. [CrossRef] [PubMed]
96. Sundqvist, G.; Carlsson, J.; Herrmann, B.; Tarnvik, A. Degradation of human immunoglobulins G and M and complement factors C3 and C5 by black-pigmented bacteroides. *J. Med. Microbiol.* **1985**, *19*, 85–94. [CrossRef] [PubMed]
97. Lina, G.; Piemont, Y.; Godail-Gamot, F.; Bes, M.; Peter, M.O.; Gauduchon, V.; Vandenesch, F.; Etienne, J. Involvement of Panton-Valentine leukocidin-producing *Staphylococcus aureus* in primary skin infections and pneumonia. *Clin. Infect. Dis.* **1999**, *29*, 1128–1132. [CrossRef]
98. Tadepalli, S.; Stewart, G.C.; Nagaraja, T.G.; Narayanan, S.K. Human *Fusobacterium necrophorum* strains have a leukotoxin gene and exhibit leukotoxic activity. *J. Med. Microbiol.* **2008**, *57*, 225–231. [CrossRef]
99. Kachlany, S.C. Aggregatibacter actinomycetemcomitans leukotoxin: From threat to therapy. *J. Dent. Res.* **2010**, *89*, 561–570. [CrossRef] [PubMed]
100. Johansson, A. *Aggregatibacter actinomycetemcomitans* leukotoxin: A powerful tool with capacity to cause imbalance in the host inflammatory response. *Toxins* **2011**, *3*, 242–259. [CrossRef] [PubMed]
101. Hoglund Aberg, C.; Kwamin, F.; Claesson, R.; Dahlen, G.; Johansson, A.; Haubek, D. Progression of attachment loss is strongly associated with presence of the JP2 genotype of *Aggregatibacter actinomycetemcomitans*: A prospective cohort study of a young adolescent population. *J. Clin. Periodontal.* **2014**, *41*, 232–241. [CrossRef]
102. Aberg, C.H.; Kelk, P.; Johansson, A. *Aggregatibacter actinomycetemcomitans*: Virulence of its leukotoxin and association with aggressive periodontitis. *Virulence* **2015**, *6*, 188–195. [CrossRef]
103. Fortanier, A.C.; Venekamp, R.P.; Boonacker, C.W.; Hak, E.; Schilder, A.G.; Sanders, E.A.; Damoiseaux, R.A. Pneumococcal conjugate vaccines for preventing acute otitis media in children. *Cochrane Database Syst. Rev.* **2019**, *5*, Cd001480. [CrossRef]
104. Wang, S.; Tafalla, M.; Hanssens, L.; Dolhain, J. A review of *Haemophilus influenzae* disease in Europe from 2000–2014: Challenges, successes and the contribution of hexavalent combination vaccines. *Expert Rev. Vaccines* **2017**, *16*, 1095–1105. [CrossRef]
105. Laine, M.L.; van Winkelhoff, A.J. Virulence of six capsular serotypes of *Porphyromonas gingivalis* in a mouse model. *Oral Microbiol. Immunol.* **1998**, *13*, 322–325. [CrossRef] [PubMed]
106. Gharbia, S.E.; Haapasalo, M.; Shah, H.N.; Kotiranta, A.; Lounatmaa, K.; Pearce, M.A.; Devine, D.A. Characterization of *Prevotella intermedia* and *Prevotella nigrescens* isolates from periodontic and endodontic infections. *J. Periodontal.* **1994**, *65*, 56–61. [CrossRef] [PubMed]
107. Singh, A.; Wyant, T.; Anaya-Bergman, C.; Aduse-Opoku, J.; Brunner, J.; Laine, M.L.; Curtis, M.A.; Lewis, J.P. The capsule of *Porphyromonas gingivalis* leads to a reduction in the host inflammatory response, evasion of phagocytosis, and increase in virulence. *Infect. Immun.* **2011**, *79*, 4533–4542. [CrossRef] [PubMed]
108. Yoshino, T.; Laine, M.L.; van Winkelhoff, A.J.; Dahlen, G. Genotype variation and capsular serotypes of *Porphyromonas gingivalis* from chronic periodontitis and periodontal abscesses. *FEMS Microbiol. Lett.* **2007**, *270*, 75–81. [CrossRef] [PubMed]
109. Slots, J. Focal infection of periodontal origin. *Periodontology 2000* **2019**, *79*, 233–235. [CrossRef] [PubMed]
110. Jepsen, S.; Caton, J.G.; Albandar, J.M.; Bissada, N.F.; Bouchard, P.; Cortellini, P.; Demirel, K.; de Sanctis, M.; Ercoli, C.; Fan, J.; et al. Periodontal manifestations of systemic diseases and developmental and acquired conditions: Consensus report of workgroup 3 of the 2017 world workshop on the classification of periodontal and peri-implant diseases and conditions. *J. Periodontal.* **2018**, *89* (Suppl. S1), S237–S248. [CrossRef] [PubMed]

111. Chen, C.K.; Wu, Y.T.; Chang, Y.C. Association between chronic periodontitis and the risk of Alzheimer's disease: A retrospective, population-based, matched-cohort study. *Alzheimers Res. Ther.* **2017**, *9*, 56. [CrossRef]
112. Potempa, J.; Mydel, P.; Koziel, J. The case for periodontitis in the pathogenesis of rheumatoid arthritis. *Nat. Rev. Rheumatol.* **2017**, *13*, 606–620. [CrossRef]
113. Konig, M.F.; Abusleme, L.; Reinholdt, J.; Palmer, R.J.; Teles, R.P.; Sampson, K.; Rosen, A.; Nigrovic, P.A.; Sokolove, J.; Giles, J.T.; et al. *Aggregatibacter actinomycetemcomitans*-induced hypercitrullination links periodontal infection to autoimmunity in rheumatoid arthritis. *Sci. Transl. Med.* **2016**, *8*, 369ra176. [CrossRef]
114. McGraw, W.T.; Potempa, J.; Farley, D.; Travis, J. Purification, characterization, and sequence analysis of a potential virulence factor from *Porphyromonas gingivalis*, peptidylarginine deiminase. *Infect. Immun.* **1999**, *67*, 3248–3256.

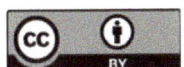 © 2019 by the authors. Licensee MDPI, Basel, Switzerland. This article is an open access article distributed under the terms and conditions of the Creative Commons Attribution (CC BY) license (http://creativecommons.org/licenses/by/4.0/).

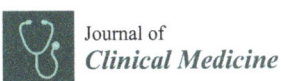

Review

Rheumatoid Arthritis-Associated Mechanisms of *Porphyromonas gingivalis* and *Aggregatibacter actinomycetemcomitans*

Eduardo Gómez-Bañuelos, Amarshi Mukherjee, Erika Darrah and Felipe Andrade *

Division of Rheumatology, The Johns Hopkins University School of Medicine, Baltimore, MD 21224, USA
* Correspondence: andrade@jhmi.edu; Tel.: +1-410-550-8665; Fax: +1-410-550-2072

Received: 30 July 2019; Accepted: 21 August 2019; Published: 26 August 2019

Abstract: Rheumatoid arthritis (RA) is an autoimmune disease of unknown etiology characterized by immune-mediated damage of synovial joints and antibodies to citrullinated antigens. Periodontal disease, a bacterial-induced inflammatory disease of the periodontium, is commonly observed in RA and has implicated periodontal pathogens as potential triggers of the disease. In particular, *Porphyromonas gingivalis* and *Aggregatibacter actinomycetemcomitans* have gained interest as microbial candidates involved in RA pathogenesis by inducing the production of citrullinated antigens. Here, we will discuss the clinical and mechanistic evidence surrounding the role of these periodontal bacteria in RA pathogenesis, which highlights a key area for the treatment and preventive interventions in RA.

Keywords: Rheumatoid arthritis; *Porphyromonas gingivalis*; *Aggregatibacter actinomycetemcomitans*; periodontitis; periodontal disease; citrullination; peptidylarginine deiminase; ACPA; anti-CCP

1. Introduction

Rheumatoid arthritis (RA) is an autoimmune disease of unknown etiology characterized by synovial inflammation, joint destruction, and high titer autoantibodies [1]. The disease affects 0.5–1% of the adult population worldwide and is associated with increased mortality rates compared with the general population [2]. A microbial origin in RA has been hypothesized for more than a century [3–6], yet, different to chronic diseases that have an infectious origin, a causal agent for RA has not been identified. Instead, numerous studies support the idea that the etiology of RA is multifactorial with a complex interplay between genetic and environmental factors [7]. Multiple risk factors have been associated with RA, including specific HLA (human leukocyte antigen) alleles, female sex, smoking, obesity, infections, and menopause, among others [8]. Nevertheless, these factors are also common in the general population, which makes it difficult to understand why only few individuals develop RA and not others with similar risk. Even in monozygotic twins, the disease concordance is rather low, varying between 8.8 and 21% [9–12]. Although stochastic events may explain the discordance in disease development among individuals at risk, the current model of RA relies on the contribution of an environmental factor, most likely a microbial agent, which may be responsible for triggering the disease in susceptible individuals.

Assuming that a microorganism is involved in RA pathogenesis, at least two hypotheses may explain why this causal agent has not yet been found. First, RA may be triggered by a rare pathogen that is exclusive to patients with RA, which has not yet been discovered because of the lack of proper technologies. Second, different to other chronic infectious diseases that are linked to a single pathogen, RA may result from the individual or interacting effects of different microbial agents likely unified by triggering common arthritogenic pathways. Moreover, like other risk factors in RA, microbial species with arthritogenic potential may also be common in the general population, but only drive RA in the perfect setting of other predisposing elements.

While it cannot be excluded that a single unknown pathogen may cause RA, current studies suggest that dysbiotic microbiomes may play a role in the pathogenesis of the disease [13–15]. In this regard, several bacterial candidates have been mechanistically linked to RA either by creating a pro-inflammatory environment or by inducing the production of autoantibodies [13–15]. Here, we will discuss the evidence surrounding the potential role of two of these microbial agents, *Porphyromonas gingivalis* (*P. gingivalis*) and *Aggregatibacter actinomycetemcomitans* (*Aa*), in the mechanistic model of RA. Importantly, these pathogens are not exclusive to RA. Indeed, they are causal agents of periodontitis, a common disease in the adult population initially associated with RA in the late 1800s [16].

2. The Focal Infection Theory, Oral Sepsis, and RA

In order to discuss the potential role of periodontal pathogens in the etiology of RA, it is important to first review the historical background leading to the link between the mouth and RA. In contrast to other arthritides known for several centuries, the first description of RA (initially termed "primary asthenic gout") was not made until 1800 by Augustin Jacob Landré-Beauvais [17]. Later, Alfred Garrod in 1859 proposed the name "rheumatoid arthritis" for diseases previously known as chronic rheumatic arthritis and rheumatic gout, and provided a detailed clinical description to distinguish RA from gout [18]. Once RA was established as an independent entity, numerous investigators tried to identify the etiology of this disease. Due to the inflammatory nature of RA, it was thought that the etiology was infectious, leading to the search for microbial organisms in the joints of patients with RA.

Between 1887 and the early 1900s, several investigators claimed to identify different bacteria in RA synovial fluid and tissue [3–6]. Although the results were inconsistent and not reproducible [19–22], these initial studies reinforced the idea that RA had an infectious origin, either due to bacteria within the joint itself or to a toxin produced by microorganisms in some other part of the body [23]. During the late 1800s, it was widely accepted that an infection in one part of the body may have effects on a different anatomical site (e.g., the syphilitic chancre is followed by systemic infection [24]). Thus, this notion fueled speculation that similar to other chronic diseases [25], RA was the result of microbial dissemination from distant sites of chronic focus of infection, including nasal sinuses, gut, lungs, genitourinary tract and the mouth [26–30]. This idea, known as the focal infection theory, defined the cause and treatment of a broad range of diseases, including RA, for several decades in the early 1900s [25,31,32].

In 1891, Willoughy D. Miller first conjectured that oral pathogens play a significant role in the production of local and systemic diseases [33,34]. This notion was further promoted by William Hunter in 1900, who was responsible for highlighting that the mouth was a major focus of infection driving diseases in other organs of the body. In particular, he reached the incorrect conclusion that pernicious anemia was the result of infective gastritis caused by oral sepsis [35–38]. Following these observations, oral sepsis (including caries, gingivitis, stomatitis, periodontitis, and tonsillitis) was considered a major focus of infection causing systemic diseases in which the etiology was unknown, such as RA [25,30,39,40]. This notion was further supported by anecdotal reports of patients with "rheumatism" cured after the removal of carious teeth [41], leading to the use of tonsillectomies and tooth extractions as the standard of treatment [29,31]. In the 1930s, this theory was refuted by the demonstration that neither tooth extraction nor tonsillectomy provided clinical benefit to patients with RA [42–44].

3. Periodontitis and RA

Among the different causes of oral sepsis that were linked to RA, an association with "pyorrhea alveolaris" was noticed in 1895 [16]. Pyorrhea alveolaris, also known as Riggs' disease and currently termed periodontal disease (PD) or periodontitis, was described by John W. Riggs in 1875 [45]. Periodontitis is a bacterial-induced chronic inflammatory disease affecting the tissues that support the teeth, including the alveolar bone. The disease results from dysbiosis of the oral microbiota and is associated with destruction of periodontal tissue, potentially leading to tooth loss [46]. Since the implantation site of the teeth is also an articulation, it was initially thought that the destruction of the periodontal membrane and alveolar bone in patients with RA and pyorrhea alveolaris was part of same RA-induced damage affecting the dentoalveolar joint [16]. Nevertheless, the establishment of the focal infection theory tilted the paradigm to underscore periodontitis as a cause (not as a consequence) of RA in the early 1900s [26–28].

However, after the downfall of the focal infection theory as the cause of RA in the 1930s, the study of periodontitis in the pathogenesis of RA was left behind. Later, at least two major advances renewed interest in periodontitis as a component of the mechanistic model of RA. The first occurred between the 1960s–1990s, when significant advances were made in the immunopathogenesis of periodontitis, which suggested important mechanistic similarities with autoimmune diseases [47], in particular RA [48]. These include common mechanisms of immune-mediated tissue damage, patterns of pro-inflammatory cytokines (e.g., interleukin (IL)-1, IL-6 and tumor necrosis factor α), immune complex deposition and complement activation [48–50]. Rapidly progressive periodontitis is also associated with *HLA-DRB1* alleles linked to RA [51,52]. Moreover, B cells and plasma cells predominate in the affected sites in chronic periodontitis [53–55], autoantibodies such as rheumatoid factor (RF) and anti-collagen antibodies are found in the periodontal lesion [56–59], and RF can be detected in dental periapical lesions from patients with RA [60]. The second advance was in 1999, when it was discovered that an important periodontal pathogen (*P. gingivalis*) secretes a peptidylarginine deiminase (PAD)-like enzyme [61], which was incorrectly thought to be equivalent to human PADs at the time [62]. As PAD enzymes are responsible for generating citrullinated proteins, major targets of autoantibodies in RA [63], it was hypothesized that periodontitis drives RA via the production of citrullinated antigens by *P. gingivalis* [62]. Together, these findings have provided the basis for the renewed theory that periodontitis and RA may be mechanistically related and potentially linked by a common etiologic factor.

In the last 10 years, numerous epidemiological studies, extensively reviewed elsewhere [64–66], have reported a positive association of RA with PD when compared to healthy (non-RA) controls. Overall, a recent meta-analysis found that patients with RA had a 13% greater risk of periodontitis compared to healthy controls, ranging from 4 to 23% (RR: 1.13; 95% CI: 1.04, 1.23; $p = 0.006$) [65]. In addition, a case-control study from the Medical Biobank of Northern Sweden found that periodontitis, characterized as marginal jawbone loss, precedes the clinical onset of RA [67], supporting a potential role for PD in RA pathogenesis. Not every study, however, has confirmed this association either by comparing RA with healthy controls [68,69] or with patients with osteoarthritis (OA) [65]. Although these studies have methodological differences that may explain their discrepancies, a causal relation between RA and periodontitis may be difficult to sustain based purely on association studies.

A major caveat in the epidemiological association between RA and periodontitis is that PD is likely the most frequent chronic infectious disease in humans worldwide. The overall rate of PD in the adult US population is 47%, with 38% over age 30 and 64% over age 65 having either severe or moderate periodontitis [70]. Moreover, severe forms of periodontitis affect 11.2% of the global adult population [71]. Considering that almost half of the adult population has some form of PD, it may be hard to demonstrate a causal relationship with RA, since its prevalence is only 0.5–1% of the adult population [2]. Indeed, the relative risk of periodontitis in patients with RA is only 1.13 when compared to healthy controls, and of 1.10 compared to OA [65]. Despite these potential shortcomings, additional studies have been centered on addressing whether periodontitis, and in particular periodontal pathogens, may have a mechanistic role in RA through the production of citrullinated antigens.

4. Citrullination and RA

The discovery that the majority of patients with RA have antibodies to citrullinated proteins (known as ACPAs) [63,72,73] marked an important advance in understanding potential pathogenic mechanisms in RA [1]. Citrullination is an enzymatic process mediated by the peptidylarginine deiminases (PADs) in which arginine residues are deiminated to generate citrulline residues [74]. Five PADs have been identified in humans (PAD1–4 and 6) [1], but only PAD1–4 have citrullinating activity [75]. PAD2 and PAD4 have gained prominence as potential candidates that drive citrullination of self-antigens in RA due to their increased expression in rheumatoid synovial tissue and fluid [76–78]. PADs are calcium dependent enzymes. Four, five, and six calcium-binding sites were identified in the structure of PAD1, PAD4, and PAD2, respectively, with calcium binding inducing conformational changes required to generate the active site cleft [79–81]. PADs are highly specific for peptidylarginine residues, requiring at least one additional amino acid residue N-terminal to the site of modification [74,82]. Thus, these enzymes can only citrullinate arginine residues within polypeptide chains but not at their termini (i.e., they are endodeiminases). Different from arginine deiminases (ADI), which catalyze the deimination of free L-arginine, PADs cannot generate citrulline from free L-arginine [74]. PADs 2, 3, and 4 form homodimers, whereas PAD1 is monomeric in solution [79–81]. Each PAD monomer contains a C-terminal catalytic domain and an N-terminal domain involved in substrate binding and protein–protein interactions [79–81]. The PADs are highly conserved and share 50%–55% sequence identity [79], but exhibit distinct substrate preferences and tissue expression [83,84].

Citrullination is a normal process across multiple tissues in humans [85]. More than 200 proteins are citrullinated in different healthy human tissues, with the highest levels found in the brain and lungs [85]. Together, this set of proteins is referred to as the citrullinome. Large amounts of citrullinated proteins are found in RA synovial fluid, including more than 100 proteins that are normally citrullinated among different normal tissues [85–91]. This unique pattern of citrullination that includes proteins spanning the range of molecular weights is termed hypercitrullination [87]. Similar to the RA joint, it is noteworthy that periodontitis is also characterized by the accumulation of large amounts of citrullinated proteins with similar patterns of hypercitrullination found in RA [92,93], supporting the notion that PD is a potential source of citrullinated autoantigens. Understanding which components in periodontitis are responsible for driving hypercitrullination may, therefore, provide important mechanistic insights into RA pathogenesis.

5. *P. gingivalis* in RA Pathogenesis

P. gingivalis was linked to periodontal disease in the early 1960s, initially named *Bacteroides melaninogenicus* (*B. melaninogenicus*) [94], which was later found to include two species, *B. melaninogenicus* (later *Prevotela melaninogenica*) and *B. asaccharolyticus* [95]. The name *B. gingivalis* was later proposed to distinguish oral from non-oral *B. asaccharolyticus* [96,97], and in the late 1980s, *B. gingivalis* was further reclassified in a new genus, the *Porphyromonas* [98]. *P. gingivalis* has been implicated in the pathogenesis of periodontitis by subverting host immune defenses, leading to overgrowth of oral commensal bacteria, which causes inflammatory tissue destruction [99,100].

Different approaches have been used to address a potential association between *P. gingivalis* and RA, many of which have shown inconsistent or inconclusive results. These include: (1) bacterial detection in gingival tissue, subgingival plaque and/or gingival crevicular fluid (GCF) either by staining using anti-*P. gingivalis* antibodies, bacterial culture, and/or DNA amplification (PCR) [101–107]; (2) metagenomic sequencing in saliva and subgingival plaque, which surveys complex microbial communities [103,106,108–112]; and (3) measuring antibodies to *P. gingivalis* in serum [101,113–125], which in contrast to the other assays that detect the existing bacteria in the mouth, it is an indirect test that determines past or present exposure to *P. gingivalis*.

Due to its convenience, the detection of antibodies to *P. gingivalis* (mainly IgG) has been the most widely used assay to study the relationship between this pathogen and RA. However, it is important to highlight that there is not a standard assay to measure such antibodies. All studies used in house ELISAs with different types of *P. gingivalis* antigens. These include bacterial cells either as intact bacteria (not fixed or fixed with formalin) or bacterial extracts generated by sonication [101,113–119], purified recombinant proteins (e.g., bacterial PAD, arginine gingipain (RgpB), or hemin binding protein 35 (HBP35)) [120–124,126], HtpG peptides (HSP90 homologue) [111], *P. gingivalis*-specific lipopolysaccharide or outer membrane antigens [125,127]. In regard to the bacterial strains, studies have included either laboratory strains or clinical isolates, which may have some antigenic differences [128]. Considering conflicting conclusions from these studies [101,113–125] and others not cited in this review, an association between anti-*P. gingivalis* antibodies and RA is difficult to sustain. However, based on a selected number of publications, two meta-analysis have reported a significant association between higher antibody titers to *P. gingivalis* and RA when compared to healthy controls with unknown PD status [129], and to healthy controls with and without PD [130]. Anti-*P. gingivalis* antibody levels also positively correlated with ACPAs in one study [129]. Nevertheless, a significant association was not found between antibodies to *P. gingivalis* and RA when compared to non-RA controls (e.g., population-based case-controls) [129]. This finding may be explained by the presence of individuals with chronic diseases and high prevalence of severe PD in the non-RA population, supporting the idea that the relative abundance of *P. gingivalis* is associated with PD severity regardless of RA [111]. Moreover, one meta-analysis showed that only antibodies to whole *P. gingivalis*, but not anti-RgpB antibodies, were positively associated with RA [129], highlighting that the anti-*P. gingivalis* antibody assays are not comparable. Interestingly, one study reported that anti-RgpB antibody concentrations increase before the onset of RA symptoms [123], suggesting a temporal relationship between *P. gingivalis* infection and the clinical onset of RA.

Unlike the detection of antibodies to *P. gingivalis*, which has shown some positive association with RA, a number of studies detecting *P. gingivalis* by PCR and metagenomic sequencing in saliva, subgingival plaque and/or GCF failed to confirm such an association [103–111]. In one of these studies, however, *P. gingivalis* was detected more frequently in a small subgroup of patients with recently diagnosed, never-treated RA, in comparison with patients with established RA or healthy controls; although this finding could be explained by a higher prevalence of severe periodontitis in those patients [111]. More recently, an increase in the relative abundance of *P. gingivalis* was found at healthy periodontal sites in at risk anti-CCP antibody positive individuals compared with anti-CCP negative healthy controls, though the significance of this finding is unclear [112].

From these studies, it is difficult to reach a definitive conclusion as to the relationship between RA and *P. ginigvalis*. A complicating factor is that every assay has different implications with regard to the status of *P. gingivalis* in the patient (e.g., carrier, active infection, or past and present exposure), and their significance is likely influenced by the source of antigen (in the case of antibodies), periodontal sample collection, and the control group used for comparison (e.g., OA, non-RA, healthy controls with or without PD). Overall, it is likely that positive associations with *P. gingivalis* may reflect PD severity rather than RA status, which importantly, neither supports nor excludes a pathogenic role for *P. gingivalis* in RA.

5.1. P. gingivalis in Experimental Models of Arthritis

In addition to epidemiological data, experimental studies using different animal models of immune-mediated arthritis (e.g., collagen-induced arthritis (CIA), methylated bovine serum albumin-induced arthritis, and the SKG mouse model) and different routes of bacterial inoculation (including oral, intraperitoneal and subcutaneous chambers) reached the conclusion that *P. gingivalis* can increase the incidence and/or exacerbate the disease [131–141].

However, many of these studies have important caveats. Several studies have reported that DBA/1 mice (a susceptible strain to induce CIA) are resistant to oral colonization by *P. gingivalis* and therefore, have recommended the use of non-oral routes of inoculation or different strains of mice to study the effect of *P. gingivalis* in experimental arthritis [131,136,142]. These findings contrast with others that have successfully induced PD with *P. gingivalis* in DBA/1 mice [132,134,135]. Among DBA/1 mice that developed periodontitis, however, there are also differences observed, with some studies showing that PD exacerbates CIA [132,134], but not others [135]. Using the SKG model of spontaneous arthritis, there are also discrepancies in the induction of PD by *P. gingivalis*, and whether this process aggravates arthritis [141,142]. Although these conflicting data may be explained by differences in mouse strains or environmental conditions that may affect the immune system in mice, the data certainly highlights the lack of reproducible mouse models to study the effect of periodontitis and P. gingivalis in autoimmune arthritis.

Using models of arthritis in rats, periodontitis induced by P. gingivalis had no effect in the development or severity of pristane-induced arthritis in Dark Agouti rats [143]. More recently, however, one study showed that P. gingivalis-associated periodontitis was sufficient to induce erosive arthritis in Lewis rats, providing the first direct evidence that P. gingivalis may have the capacity to induce arthritis [144].

Several mechanisms have been proposed by which P. gingivalis may promote autoimmune arthritis in humans and in experimental animals. These include the induction of a systemic Th17 cell response [132–134], induction of autoantibodies [131,138,143,144], cross-reactivity between bacterial and host antigens [145], by promoting C5a generation [141], through direct dissemination of P. gingivalis into the joints [136], and by swallowing the bacteria, which may alter the gut microbiota and gut immune system [137]. Nevertheless, the production of citrullinated autoantigens by a PAD enzyme released from P. gingivalis is considered the most important mechanistic evidence to support a role of P. gingivalis in RA pathogenesis [14,146].

5.2. P. gingivalis PAD (PPAD)

The existence of an arginine deiminase-like enzyme in P. gingivalis was suggested in the early 1990's [147], and the enzyme was purified and characterized in 1999 [61]. PPAD is not evolutionarily related to mammalian PADs. Structurally, it is a close relative of agmatine deiminases, which are found across bacteria [148]. Different to mammalian PADs, PPAD does not require calcium for catalysis, it is only composed of a ~40 kDa catalytic domain, and it can convert free L-arginine to free L-citrulline [61,148,149]. In addition, PPAD only modifies C-terminal arginine residues (i.e., an exodeiminase), as those generated after peptide cleavage by arginine gingipain (Rgp) [149], which is also secreted by P. gingivalis. Several PPAD variants have been identified through the analysis of P. gingivalis genomes and clinical isolates [150]. One of these variants (termed PPAD-T2) has two-fold higher catalytic activity compared with PPAD from the reference strain (PPAD-T1) [150]. Whether PPAD variants are relevant for P. gingivalis pathogenesis is unknown.

PPAD is detected in the outer membrane (OM) fractions of P. gingivalis and as a secreted enzyme, which is found in a soluble form and in association with outer membrane vesicles (OMVs) [120,151,152]. In most clinical isolates (termed type I isolates), extracellular PPAD is mainly found in secreted OMVs and to a minor extent in a soluble form. In contrast, a small subset of clinical isolates (termed type II isolates) showed minimal levels of PPAD in OMVs and most of the enzyme in the soluble form [152]. Type II isolates are associated with a lysine residue at position 373 in PPAD [152]. The clinical significance of P. gingivalis type I and type II subsets in the pathogenesis of PD and RA is unknown. Secreted PPAD is believed to be a major virulence factor of P. gingivalis due to its capacity to generate ammonia during deimination of arginine to citrulline. Ammonia may protect P. gingivalis during acidic cleansing in the mouth [153], and promote periodontal infection by inhibiting neutrophil function [154,155].

5.3. PPAD-Mediated Citrullination of Bacterial and Host Proteins

A potential association between PPAD and citrullination in RA was initially suggested as a hypothesis in 2004 [62]. The first experimental evidence, published in 2010, provided two major findings [156]. The first was that clinical isolates of P. gingivalis were highly enriched in citrullinated proteins, suggesting that Rgp and PPAD are actively cleaving and citrullinating a large number of substrates in P. gingivalis. The second was that after cleavage by Rgp, PPAD citrullinates C-terminal arginine residues in fibrinogen and α-enolase, two important targets of ACPAs in RA. Together, these data provided initial evidence to suggest that bacterial and host proteins citrullinated by PPAD might initiate the loss of tolerance to citrullinated autoantigens in RA [156].

Subsequent studies, however, did not confirm the abundant citrullination initially found in *P. gingivalis* [120,128]. Indeed, although PPAD may citrullinate some proteins in *P. gingivalis*, this feature appears to be exclusive to a few bacterial strains (it was only detectable in reference strain W83 and the clinical isolate MDS45), and potential citrullination seems to be limited to only six bacterial proteins [128]. Whether C-terminal citrullinated peptides derived from these bacterial proteins are specific targets of ACPAs is unknown. Interestingly, PPAD is stable at low pH, resistant to limited proteolysis, and retains significant activity after boiling [61]. Therefore, depending on the processing of *P. gingivalis* for protein analysis, it is possible that citrullination of bacterial proteins may occur in vitro following cell lysis [120]. As an artifact, this may explain the reports of abundant citrullination (including endocitrullination) in lysates from *P. gingivalis* [121,157], as well as the finding that some monoclonal ACPAs cross-react with citrullinated outer membrane antigens (OMAs) from *P. gingivalis* lysates [157].

Regarding autoantigen citrullination by *P. gingivalis* [156], it is important to highlight that neither Rgp nor PPAD have substrate specificity. The finding that fibrinogen and α-enolase are cleaved and citrullinated by these enzymes is, therefore, not surprising, as any other protein would be predicted to undergo the same processing when exposed to these enzymes. Since cleavage and citrullination by Rgp and PPAD is not specific for RA autoantigens, additional evidence is required to support a role of PPAD in the lack of tolerance to citrullinated autoantigens. For example, this could be achieved by demonstrating that C-terminal citrullination mediated by Rgp and PPAD enhances immunoreactivity to autoantigens in RA.

5.4. Self-Endocitrullination of Pro-PPAD

PPAD is expressed as a pro-enzyme (thereafter pro-PPAD) that contains four domains: an N-terminal pro-peptide, a catalytic domain, an immunoglobulin-superfamily (IgSF) domain and a C-terminal domain (CTD) [148,149]. The mature enzyme only contains the catalytic and IgSF domains [148]. N-terminal processing appears to maintain enzyme activity and stability [120,158], while C-terminal cleavage is required for cell surface translocation of PPAD [159,160]. During the production and immunogenic analysis of recombinant pro-PPAD, it was noticed that the pro-enzyme undergoes self-endocitrullination when expressed in *E. coli*, and that this modified protein was preferentially recognized by RA sera when compared with the native pro-enzyme [121]. Using 13 cyclic PPAD peptides (termed CPP1-CPP13, which should not be confused with cyclic citrullinated peptides or CCPs) encompassing 18 potential citrullination sites in pro-PPAD, the study further identified immunodominant endocitrullinated peptides recognized by RA antibodies [121]. Although these results were surprising, because PPAD has no endocitrullination activity, it was assumed that these findings were analogous to PPAD from *P. gingivalis*. Thus, the data were interpreted to suggest that loss of tolerance to citrullinated proteins in RA may originate from an antimicrobial immune response directed against citrullinated PPAD [121].

Nevertheless, further studies demonstrated that self-endocitrullination of pro-PPAD was an artifact that resulted from the lack of N-terminal processing of the enzyme expressed in *E. coli* [120]. The absence of endocitrullination in PPAD has been additionally confirmed in structural studies using processed PPAD expressed in *E. coli* or generated in *P. gingivalis* [148,149]. In accordance with these findings, it was also demonstrated that although patients with RA have antibodies to PPAD, these antibodies have no preferential reactivity to the citrullinated pro-enzyme made in *E. coli* [120]. Together, these data demonstrated that self-endocitrullination of pro-PPAD in *E. coli* and the serum reactivity to this modified protein are unlikely to reflect the function and immunogenicity of PPAD from *P. gingivalis* [14,120,161].

Although some RA sera appear to react with cyclic citrullinated peptides derived from pro-PPAD (i.e., CPPs) [121,162], it is unclear whether these peptides are recognized by antibodies to native PPAD or if similar to commercial CCPs, CPPs may function as non-specific targets to detect ACPAs [161]. In this regard, although it was justified that CPPs were generated without knowledge that endocitrullination of pro-PPAD in *E. coli* was an artifact, there is no scientific support to continue their use in the study of RA. Nevertheless, antibodies to CPPs are still being used as biomarkers to link PPAD self-endocitrullination and RA pathogenesis. In particular, serum reactivity against the peptide termed CPP3 has been used to define clinical associations between *P. gingivalis* and RA [122,123,163,164], and to demonstrate that *P. gingivalis* can induce antibodies to citrullinated PPAD in rats [143]. Since the significance of CPPs is unclear, the findings generated with these peptides should be taken with caution. More importantly, serum reactivity to CPPs should not be considered as a maker of citrullination induced by PPAD.

5.5. PPAD in Experimental Models of Arthritis

To establish a direct role of PPAD in the production of ACPAs in RA, several experimental models of arthritis have been used to demonstrate that *P. gingivalis* induces or exacerbates arthritis *via* PPAD-mediated autoantigen citrullination and ACPA production. However, while several studies appear to confirm this hypothesis [131,138,144], these studies also highlight important misunderstandings in the study of protein citrullination and ACPAs in RA. For example, in a model of *P. gingivalis* and CIA, citrullinated proteins were mistakenly quantified by a colorimetric method, which measures both free citrulline and peptidylcitrulline [131]. In addition, unconventional methods have been used to detect or define ACPAs. This include the quantification of IgG levels against ACPA (i.e., anti-ACPA antibodies) rather than antibodies to the citrullinated substrates themselves [138]. More recently, one study showed that *P. gingivalis* drives ACPAs (detected by the anti-CCP2 assay) and erosive arthritis in Lewis rats, providing the first evidence that this microbial agent may be arthritogenic [144]. However, it also demonstrated that the antibody response was not specific to the citrullinated forms of antigens [144].

The failure to demonstrate a role of PPAD in autoantigen citrullination and ACPA production in mice and rats is not surprising. Although these animal models express synovial citrullinated proteins and recapitulate several features of the human disease [140,165], they do not produce antibodies specific for citrullinated proteins as observed in RA [165–169]. Moreover, they have a high amount of false-positive reactivity toward citrullinated peptides [166], which is frequently misinterpreted as ACPA positivity when non-citrullinated peptide controls are not included to confirm specificity [131,139,140]. Considering these important shortcomings, even if PPAD plays a critical role in the induction of ACPAs in RA, this hypothesis will be hard to demonstrate using current models of immune-mediated arthritis. Indeed, the data from some animal models of arthritis strongly suggest that *P. gingivalis* may exacerbate or induce disease by mechanisms independent of ACPA production, which may involve the activity of PPAD as a virulence factor targeting either free L-citrulline or protein substrates [131]. Thus, although epidemiological and experimental data may suggest a potential role of *P. gingivalis* in RA pathogenesis, there is no experimental evidence to support that this process is mediated by the induction of ACPAs against host or bacterial proteins citrullinated by PPAD.

6. *Aa* in RA Pathogenesis

6.1. Infection Due to Aa

Aa, initially named *Bacterium actinomycetem comitans*, is a Gram-negative oral pathobiont first described in 1912 as a co-isolate from actinomycosis lesions [170]. It was reclassified as *Actinobacillus actinomycetemcomitans* and *Haemophilus actinomycetemcomitans* [171], and finally transferred in 2006 to a new genus, the *Aggregatibacter* [172]. For many years, it was thought that *Aa* was unable to cause infection, except in conjunction with *Actinomyces* [173,174]. This idea was initially supported by the finding that injection of a pure culture of *Aa* in the skin of a normal individual produced no infection [174]. In the 1960's, however, several cases of *Aa* infection not associated with actinomycosis were reported, which were mainly associated with endocarditis [175–177]. *Aa* is now considered part of the HACEK (*Haemophilus, Aggregatibacter* (previously *Actinobacillus*), *Cardiobacterium, Eikenella, Kingella*) group of bacteria that are an unusual cause of infective endocarditis [178]. In addition, it is recognized as a cause of serious infections that can affect almost any organ, although these are very uncommon [179,180].

Although *Aa* is a rare cause of infection, this bacterium has attracted special attention since the 1980s because of its strong association with severe forms of periodontitis [181–185], both localized aggressive periodontitis (LAP) and chronic periodontitis [181,182,186–195]. *Aa* expresses several virulence factors [196]. Among these, the production of leukotoxin A (LtxA) is considered the major pathogenic component in the progression of aggressive periodontitis [195]. LtxA is a member of the repeats-in-toxin (RTX) family of pore-forming proteins [197]. Lymphocyte function-associated antigen (LFA)-1 (CD11a/CD18), Mac-1 (CD11b/CD18) and $\alpha_X\beta_2$ (CD11c/CD18) act as receptors for LtxA (CD18 harbors the major binding site for LtxA), which accounts for the selective killing of human leukocytes [198]. By secreting LtxA, *Aa* induces cytolysis of target cells, thereby disabling host immune defenses and permitting escape from immune surveillance. *Aa* isolates exhibit variable virulence potential [195]. Strains of the serotype b JP2 genotype, characterized by a 530-bp deletion in the promoter region of the leukotoxin operon, has been shown to be highly virulent [199,200]. This genotype, which expresses 10- to 20-fold-higher levels of LtxA due to deletion of a transcriptional terminator [201], is associated with LAP primarily in subjects of African descent [202]. A more detailed analysis of the pathogenic mechanisms associated with the induction of periodontitis by *Aa* have been reviewed recently. [203]

6.2. Aa-Induced Hypercitrullination and the Production Citrullinated RA Autoantigens

A role of *Aa* in the pathogenesis of RA was suggested in 2016, during the search for periodontal pathogens that may explain the presence of hypercitrullination in periodontitis [92]. The study of gingival tissue from patients with PD using anti-citrulline antibodies provided initial evidence that protein citrullination is increased in PD [204,205], supporting the idea that periodontitis is a potential source of citrullinated autoantigens. In addition, the data suggested the possibility that this process was linked to the activity of PPAD [205]. However, although further analysis by mass spectrometry (MS) of GCF confirmed that protein citrullination is increased in PD, this approach also provided two novel findings [92]. First, GCF from patients with PD is highly enriched in citrullinated proteins, mimicking patterns of cellular hypercitrullination found in the rheumatoid joint [92]. Second, peptide spectra of citrullinated proteins in periodontitis were consistent with endocitrullination [92], suggesting that an abnormal activation of host PADs, rather than PPAD, may be responsible for this process. Importantly, the presence of endocitrullination in periodontitis has been further confirmed by MS in GCF and periodontal tissue from patients with PD, both with and without RA [93].

Among different microbial species associated with severe periodontitis, in vitro studies identified *Aa* as the only pathogen that could reproduce the citrullinome found in periodontitis and RA, including the production of well-known targets of ACPAs [92]. In contrast to *P. gingivalis*, however, *Aa* does not encode a PAD-like enzyme. Instead, *Aa* drives citrullination by hyperactivating host PADs through the activity of LtxA. This toxin targets neutrophils, which are enriched in PAD enzymes and constitute the major immune cells in PD and the RA joint [206–208]. Since PADs are calcium dependent, the prominent calcium influx generated by the lytic effect of LtxA hyperactivates these enzymes, driving global hypercitrullination of a wide range of cellular proteins [92]. During this process, cell membrane integrity is eventually lost and membrane rupture occurs with release of citrullinated contents into the extracellular space [92]. Interestingly, this process is similar to the induction of hypercitrullination by host immune-effector pathways (i.e., perforin and complement) in the RA joint [87], suggesting that membranolytic damage by pore-forming proteins may be a unifying mechanism in the production of citrullinated autoantigens [209]. The form of cell death induced by these pore-forming mechanisms has recently been named leukotoxic hypercitrullination (LTH) [209], to distinguish it from other forms of neutrophil death that do not induce hypercitrullination.

6.3. Aa Exposure and RA Pathogenesis

Similar to *P. gingivalis*, epidemiological studies to identify an association between *Aa* and RA have been done by detecting antibodies in serum. In particular, IgG antibodies to LtxA (used as markers of *Aa* infection) have been measured in two large cohorts of patients with RA [92,210]. In one study that included patients with established RA, anti-LtxA antibodies were significantly associated with RA when compared to healthy individuals without PD [92]. Similarly, anti-LtxA antibodies were associated with chronic periodontitis in patients without RA, and the strongest association was observed in individuals with severe periodontitis [92]. Antibodies to LtxA may, therefore, identify a subgroup of RA patients with moderate to severe PD. Interestingly, this study also found that the association between *HLA-DRB1* susceptibility alleles (known as shared epitope alleles) and RA autoantibodies was restricted to patients who had evidence of *Aa* exposure. This suggested that in susceptible individuals, LtxA-induced hypercitrullination may play a role in ACPA production [92]. In support of this hypothesis, ACPA production and RA-like symptoms were recently reported in a patient with *Aa* endocarditis who had strong a genetic susceptibility to RA conferred by three HLA alleles linked to ACPA-positive RA [211].

In a different study using a large cohort of patients with early RA, anti-LtxA antibodies were also significantly enriched in RA compared to healthy controls and patients with other inflammatory arthritides (in both groups PD status was unknown) [210], supporting the high prevalence of *Aa* exposure in RA, both in early and established disease. However, this study found that the interaction between *HLA-DRB1*-SE and anti-CCP positivity was not exclusive to anti-LtxA-positive patients with RA [210]. Major differences among these cohorts may explain this discrepancy [212].

Analogous to *P. gingivalis*, metagenomic sequencing and PCR analysis in subgingival plaque have not found a significant association between the presence of *Aa* and RA [104,105,108,110]. In one study, however, analysis of GCF using commercial DNA probes (micro-Ident) identified *Aa* as the only periodontal pathogen showing significant differences between RA and non-RA controls (both with and without PD) [107]. Thus, similar to *P. gingivalis*, positive associations with *Aa* likely indicate PD severity irrespective of RA status.

Few studies have explored the potential role of *Aa* in experimental arthritis [142,213]. However, defining the causal effect of *Aa* in animal models of arthritis has the same limitations as those described for the study of *P. gingivalis*. Moreover, LtxA is known to have activity against leukocytes in primates, with no toxicity on rodent cells [214]. Therefore, different to the human model, any effect that *Aa* may have in the induction of experimental arthritis in rodents is unlikely to be driven by LtxA-induced hypercitrullination and the production of ACPAs.

7. *P. gingivalis* and *Aa* in the Mechanistic Model of RA: Causal Agents, Risk Factors, Disease Modulators, or Research Distractors

Assuming that periodontitis has a mechanistic role in RA, *P. gingivalis* and *Aa* may influence disease pathogenesis at different phases of RA development. The production of autoantibodies is an early and asymptomatic event that precedes the clinical onset of RA by several years [215,216]. The presence of a chronic and amplifying immune response against bacterial-induced RA autoantigens, in particular citrullinated antigens is, therefore, one of the most attractive hypothesis to explain disease initiation and potentially a causal association. In this context, this model explains why there is so much interest in establishing a causal relationship between *P. gingivalis* and the production of ACPAs in either experimental arthritis or RA. Although the current evidence neither demonstrate nor exclude the possibility that PPAD generates citrullinated autoantigens, other possibilities may explain a potential role of *P. gingivalis* in RA pathogenesis. Interestingly, protein citrullination is a process that is increased during inflammation [217]. However, while transient inflammation may not be sufficient to initiate an immune response to citrullinated proteins, periodontitis is a chronic non-fatal illnesses that can start during adolescence and progress over decades [218]. During this time, it is possible that some individuals at risk may develop autoantibodies to citrullinated proteins. *P. gingivalis*, a keystone microorganism in periodontitis, is certainly a strong candidate for promoting chronic inflammation [100], which may indirectly drive the production of autoantibodies in susceptible individuals.

In contrast to *P. gingivalis*, a potential role of *Aa* in the lack of tolerance to RA-associated autoantigens involves the induction of lytic hypercitrullination [92]. In this regard, different factors such as *Aa* virulence (i.e., LtxA production) and bacterial load may define the risk of developing autoantibodies in the context of *Aa* infection in susceptible individuals [92,211]. Importantly, as other bacterial species also produce pore-forming toxins [219], it is possible that other pathogens may induce hypercitrullination and ACPAs at other mucosal sites, including the lung and gut [1,209]. LTH as a mechanism of autoantigen production by different pathogens may explain why every patient with seropositive RA does not have exposure to *Aa* and/or PD.

Interestingly, patients with RA show abnormalities in central and peripheral B cell tolerance checkpoints [220–222], likely due to an intrinsic genetic predisposition [223,224]. This results in the accumulation of autoreactive and polyreactive B cells that can recognize immunoglobulins and citrullinated peptides [220,221]. Depending on genetic and environmental risk factors, autoreactive or polyreactive naïve B cells may have a selective advantage to develop into high affinity autoreactive memory B cells through somatic mutations and affinity maturation. In this scenario, autoantigens generated by arthritogenic bacteria may promote the expansion and maturation of already existing autoreactive cells, rather than initiating the loss of tolerance to host antigens. A prerequisite of having autoreactive/polyreactive B cells to induce pathogenic autoantibodies by *P. gingivalis* or *Aa* may explain why only a limited number of individuals with PD may develop RA.

Although the hypothesis that periodontal pathogens (e.g., *P. gingivalis* or *Aa*) are causal agents of RA is an attractive idea, it is also possible that these bacteria may only be relevant as risk factors for the development of ACPA-positive RA. Alternatively, once RA has been established, persistent low-grade inflammation associated with PD may modulate RA progression and severity. Lastly, despite the enormous enthusiasm of demonstrating that periodontitis is relevant for RA pathogenesis, it cannot yet be excluded that patients with RA may have a higher risk of developing PD (even during the pre-clinical phase of RA), but neither periodontitis, *P. gingivalis*, nor *Aa* may play a pathogenic role in the disease.

8. Therapeutic Implications

The possibility of identifying a factor that triggers a multifactorial disease, such as RA, has critical implications for treatment and preventive interventions. The success of any therapy, however, may depend on targeting such a factor at the correct time during the evolution of the disease [225]. In this regard, although a systematic review and meta-analysis suggested that periodontal treatment may decrease some markers of disease activity in RA [226], these findings remain controversial [227]. The lack of an efficient response to PD treatment on RA disease activity may suggest that periodontitis has no pathogenic role in RA, or that it is most important for disease initiation, during the pre-clinical phase, and that treatment during established disease is no longer effective. If a periodontal pathogen is relevant for the initial breech of tolerance to arthritogenic autoantigens, aiming to treat asymptomatic autoantibody positive (e.g., anti-CCP, RF, or any other autoantibody) individuals may still be too late to stop the progression to symptomatic RA. In this scenario, preventive therapies (e.g., oral hygiene and potentially vaccines against periodontal pathogens) should be initiated in at-risk individuals prior to the development of these serologies. In contrast, if periodontitis is important for the amplification of the autoimmune response in preclinical RA, there is a window of opportunity to target seropositive asymptomatic individuals. Indeed, to date, this is the most feasible hypothesis that could be therapeutically addressed. However, if periodontal pathogens only play a role in the induction of specific subtypes of autoantibodies (e.g., ACPAs), eradication of these agents during the pre-clinical phase of the disease may only decrease the risk of developing certain autoantibodies (and potentially further RA severity), but may not change the course of the disease, including the production of antibodies to other autoantigens. Interestingly, recent evidence suggest that periodontitis is a potential source of proteins modified by malondialdehyde-acetaldehyde adducts and carbamylation [228], which are also common targets of autoantibodies in RA. [229] Thus, independent of the periodontal pathogen, preventing, or targeting periodontitis may be the best exploratory option to prevent RA.

9. Conclusions

Although some epidemiological and mechanistic data supports a role for *P. gingivalis* and *Aa* in the pathogenic model of RA, it is important to underscore that these oral pathobionts do not fulfill the Henle-Koch's postulates of causation [230–232]. These microbial agents neither occur in every case of the disease, nor are specific for patients with RA. In the context of inducing ACPA production in vivo to satisfy the third postulate, it will require the use of animal models that can truly reproduce the autoantibody response observed in RA. Considering these shortcomings, demonstrating or discarding a role of *P. gingivalis* and *Aa* in the pathogenesis of RA may require a different view of how to define disease causality by these microbial agents [212].

In the case of *P. gingivalis*, it is imperative to recognize that its potential role in RA involves elucidation of at least three different questions. The first is whether *P. gingivalis* is relevant for RA pathogenesis, either by initiating or exacerbating the disease. The second is whether *P. gingivalis* is important for RA because of the production of PPAD or because it plays a critical role in the induction of periodontitis by inciting inflammation. Indeed, it appears that ligation-induced periodontitis (without additional infection with *P. gingivalis*) is sufficient to exacerbate CIA in Wistar rats [233]. The third is whether PPAD drives RA due to the production of citrullinated antigens and the induction of ACPAs in the host or because this enzyme is a virulence factor that facilitates bacterial growth and the establishment of PD. Although these questions have been somewhat addressed, definitive conclusions cannot be reached from the available data. Defining the role of PPAD in the production of citrullinated antigens and whether C-terminal deimination offers an advantage for peptide immunogenicity remains a high priority. Importantly, other potential arthritogenic mechanisms induced by *P. gingivalis*, besides autoantigen citrullination, should be kept in consideration.

In the case of *Aa*, this model offers an advantage over other periodontal bacteria because of its capacity to induce neutrophil hypercitrullination and the release of citrullinated autoantigens through osmotic lysis [92]. However, the number of studies linking *Aa* with RA are too limited to truly determine its pathogenic significance for the disease. Similar to *P. gingivalis*, rigorous studies are necessary to support or refute the role of *Aa* in the etiology of RA. Together, these oral pathobionts pose an opportunity to understand whether bacterial-associated citrullination is a mechanism involved in RA pathogenesis. This has important implications for the implementation of preventive interventions in RA.

Author Contributions: Conceptualization and writing—original draft preparation: F.A.; writing—review and editing: E.G.-B., A.M., and E.D.

Funding: This research was funded by the Jerome L. Greene Foundation, Rheumatology Research Foundation, and National Institute of Arthritis and Musculoskeletal and Skin Diseases (NIAMS) at the National Institutes of Health (NIH) grant number R01 AR069569. The content of this paper is solely the responsibility of the author and does not represent the official views of the NIAMS or the NIH.

Conflicts of Interest: F.A. and E.D. are authors on issued patent no. 8,975,033, entitled "Human autoantibodies specific for PAD3 which are cross-reactive with PAD4 and their use in the diagnosis and treatment of rheumatoid arthritis and related diseases" and on provisional patent no. 62/481,158 entitled "Anti-PAD2 antibody for treating and evaluating rheumatoid arthritis". F.A. serves as consultant for Bristol-Myers Squibb. E.D. received a research grant from Pfizer and from Bristol-Myers Squibb. E.D. previously served on the scientific advisory board for Padlock Therapeutics, Inc. The remaining authors declare that they have no conflicts of interests.

References

1. Darrah, E.; Andrade, F. Rheumatoid arthritis and citrullination. *Curr. Opin. Rheumatol.* **2018**, *30*, 72–78. [CrossRef]

2. Carmona, L.; Cross, M.; Williams, B.; Lassere, M.; March, L. Rheumatoid arthritis. *Best Pract. Res. Clin. Rheumatol.* **2010**, *24*, 733–745. [CrossRef] [PubMed]
3. Mantle, A. The etiology of rheumatism considered from a bacterial point of view. *Br. Med. J.* **1887**, *1*, 1381–1384. [CrossRef] [PubMed]
4. Bannatyne, G.A.; Wohlmann, A.S.; Blaxall, F.R. Rheumatoid arthritis: Its clinical history, etiology, and pathology. *Lancet* **1896**, *147*, 1120–1125. [CrossRef]
5. Schuller, M. The relation of chronic villous polyarthritis to the dumb-bell shaped bacilli. *Am. J. Med. Sci.* **1906**, *132*, 231–239. [CrossRef]
6. Schuller, M. Chirurgische Mittheilungen über die Chronisch-Rheumatischen Glenkentzündungen. In *Archiv Fur Klinische Chirurgie*; Bergman, E.V., Billroth, T., Gurlt, E., Eds.; Verlag Von August Hirschwald: Berlin, Germany, 1893; pp. 153–185.
7. McInnes, I.B.; Schett, G. The Pathogenesis of Rheumatoid Arthritis. *N. Engl. J. Med.* **2011**, *365*, 2205–2219. [CrossRef] [PubMed]
8. Deane, K.D.; Demoruelle, M.K.; Kelmenson, L.B.; Kuhn, K.A.; Norris, J.M.; Holers, V.M. Genetic and environmental risk factors for rheumatoid arthritis. *Best Pract. Res. Clin. Rheumatol.* **2017**, *31*, 3–18. [CrossRef] [PubMed]
9. Svendsen, A.J.; Kyvik, K.O.; Houen, G.; Junker, P.; Christensen, K.; Christiansen, L.; Nielsen, C.; Skytthe, A.; Hjelmborg, J.V. On the Origin of Rheumatoid Arthritis: The Impact of Environment and Genes—A Population Based Twin Study. *PLoS ONE* **2013**, *8*, e57304. [CrossRef] [PubMed]
10. Frisell, T.; Saevarsdottir, S.; Askling, J.; Frisell, T. Family history of rheumatoid arthritis: An old concept with new developments. *Nat. Rev. Rheumatol.* **2016**, *12*, 335–343. [CrossRef] [PubMed]
11. Silman, A.J.; MacGregor, A.J.; Thomson, W.; Holligan, S.; Carthy, D.; Farhan, A.; Ollier, W.E.R. Twin concordance rates for rheumatoid arthritis: Results from a nationwide study. *Br. J. Rheumatol.* **1993**, *32*, 903–907. [CrossRef] [PubMed]
12. Svendsen, A.J.; Holm, N.V.; Kyvik, K.; Petersen, P.H.; Junker, P. Relative importance of genetic effects in rheumatoid arthritis: Historical cohort study of Danish nationwide twin population. *BMJ* **2002**, *324*, 264. [CrossRef] [PubMed]
13. Caminer, A.C.; Haberman, R.; Scher, J.U. Human microbiome, infections, and rheumatic disease. *Clin. Rheumatol.* **2017**, *36*, 2645–2653. [CrossRef] [PubMed]
14. Potempa, J.; Mydel, P.; Koziel, J. The case for periodontitis in the pathogenesis of rheumatoid arthritis. *Nat. Rev. Rheumatol.* **2017**, *13*, 606–620. [CrossRef] [PubMed]
15. Scher, J.U.; Littman, D.R.; Abramson, S.B. Microbiome in Inflammatory Arthritis and Human Rheumatic Diseases. *Arthritis Rheumatol.* **2016**, *68*, 35–45. [CrossRef] [PubMed]
16. Dunbar, L.L. Oral manifestations in arthritic and gouty conditions. *JAMA* **1895**, *24*, 75–77. [CrossRef]
17. Landré-Beauvais, A.J. The first description of rheumatoid arthritis. Unabridged text of the doctoral dissertation presented in 1800. *Jt. Bone Spine* **2001**, *68*, 130–143.
18. Garrod, A.B. Rheumatic Gout. In *The Nature and Treatment of Gout and Rheumatic Gout*; Garrod, A.B., Ed.; Walton and Maberly: London, UK, 1859; pp. 526–556.
19. Richards, J.H. Bacteriologic Studies in Chronic Arthritis and Chorea. *J. Bacteriol.* **1920**, *5*, 511–525. [PubMed]
20. Swett, P.P. Synovectomy in chronic infectious arthritis. *J. Bone Jt. Surg.* **1923**, *5*, 110–121.
21. Kinsella, R.A. Chronic infectious arthritis. *J. Am. Med. Assoc.* **1923**, *80*, 0671–0674. [CrossRef]
22. Margolis, M.H.; Dorsey, A.H.E. Chronic arthritis—Bacteriology of affected tissues. *Arch. Intern. Med.* **1930**, *46*, 121–136. [CrossRef]
23. Goadby, K.W. The Hunterian Lecture on the Association of Disease of the Mouth with Rheumatoid Arthritis and Certain other Forms of Rheumatism. Delivered at the Royal College of Surgeons of England on March 6th, 1911. *Lancet* **1911**, *1*, 639–649.
24. Lane, S.A. A Lecture on Tertiary Syphilis, or Syphilitic Cachexia. *Br. Med. J.* **1873**, *2*, 421–423. [CrossRef] [PubMed]
25. Billings, I.K. Focal infection—Its broader application in the etiology of general disease. *J. Am. Med. Assoc.* **1914**, *63*, 899–903. [CrossRef]
26. Lambert, J. A report of some points in the etiology and onset of 195 cases of rheumatoid arthritis. *Bull. Comm. Study Spec. Dis.* **1908**, *2*, 83–94.
27. Lindsay, J. The relation of infective foci to rheumatoid arthritis. *Bull. Comm. Study Spec. Dis.* **1908**, *2*, 106–116.

28. Billings, F. Chronic focal infections and their etiologic relations to arthritis and nephritis. *Arch. Intern. Med.* **1912**, *9*, 484–498. [CrossRef]
29. Billings, F. Chronic focal infection as a causative factor in chronic arthritis. *J. Am. Med. Assoc.* **1913**, *61*, 819–822. [CrossRef]
30. Billings, F. Mouth infection as a source of systemic disease. *J. Am. Med. Assoc.* **1914**, *63*, 2024–2025. [CrossRef]
31. Bywaters, E.G.L. Historical Aspects of the Aetiology of Rheumatoid Arthritis. *Br. J. Rheumatol.* **1988**, 110–115. [CrossRef]
32. Hughes, R.A. Focal infection revisited. *Br. J. Rheumatol.* **1994**, *33*, 370–377. [CrossRef]
33. Miller, W.D. The Human Mouth as a Focus of Infection. *Dent. Cosmos.* **1891**, *33*, 689–713. [CrossRef]
34. Miller, W.D. Diseases of the Human Body Which Have Been Traced to the Action of Mouth-Bacteria. *Am. J. Dent. Sci.* **1891**, *25*, 311–319. [PubMed]
35. Hunter, W. Oral Sepsis as a Cause of Disease. *Br. Med. J.* **1900**, *2*, 215–216. [CrossRef] [PubMed]
36. Hunter, W. A Case of Pernicious Anæmia; with Observations regarding Mode of Onset, Clinical Features, Infective Nature, Prognosis, and Antiseptic and Serum Treatment of the Disease. *J. R. Soc. Med.* **1901**, *84*, 205–249.
37. Hunter, W. Further observations on pernicious anaemia (seven cases): A chronic infective disease; its relation to infection from the mouth and stomach; suggested serum treatment. *Lancet* **1900**, *155*, 296–299. [CrossRef]
38. Hunter, W. Further investigations regarding the infective nature and etiology of pernicius anaemia. *Lancet* **1903**, *161*, 367–371. [CrossRef]
39. Roberts, H.L. Focal infection. *Br. J. Derm. Syph.* **1921**, *33*, 319–334. [CrossRef]
40. Roberts, H.L. Focal infection. *Br. J. Derm. Syph.* **1921**, *33*, 353–373. [CrossRef]
41. Rush, B. An Account of the Cure of Several Diseases by the Extraction of Decayed Teeth. In *Medical Inquiries and Observations*, 5th ed.; Rush, B., Ed.; Printed by M. Carey & Son; B. Warner; A. Finley; S. W. Conrad; T. & W. Bradford; B. & T. Kite, and Bennett and Walton; National Library of Medicine: Philadelphia, PA, USA, 1818; Volume 1, pp. 197–201. Available online: https://collections.nlm.nih.gov/catalog/nlm:nlmuid-2569006RX1-mvpart (accessed on 26 August 2019).
42. Miltner, L.J.; Kulowski, J. The effect of treatment and erradication of foci on infection in chronic rheumatoid arthritis. *J. Bone Jt. Surg.* **1933**, *15*, 383–396.
43. Cecil, R.; Angevine, A. Clinical and experimental observations on focal infection. *Ann. Intern. Med.* **1938**, *12*, 577–584.
44. Vaizey, J.M.; Clark-Kennedy, A.E. Dental Sepsis: Anaemia, Dyspepsia, and Rheumatism. *Br. Med. J.* **1939**, *1*, 1269–1273. [CrossRef]
45. Riggs, J.W. Suppurative Inflammation of the Gums and Absorption of the Gums and the Alveolar Process. *Am. J. Dent. Sci.* **1999**, *32*, 401–407.
46. Hajishengallis, G. Immunomicrobial pathogenesis of periodontitis: Keystones, pathobionts, and host response. *Trends Immunol.* **2014**, *35*, 3–11. [CrossRef]
47. Brandtzaeg, P.; Kraus, F.W. Autoimmunity and periodontal disease. *Odontol. Tidskr.* **1965**, *73*, 281.
48. Snyderman, R.; McCarty, G.A. Analogous Mechanisms of Tissue Destruction in Rheumatoid Arthritis and Periodontal Disease. In *Host-Parasite Interactions in Periodontal Diseases*; Genco, R.J., Mergenhagen, S.E., Eds.; American Society of Microbiology: Washington, DC, USA, 1982; pp. 354–362.
49. Seymour, G.J.; Powell, R.N.; Davies, W.I.R. The immunopathogenesis of progressive chronic inflammatory periodontal disease. *J. Oral. Pathol. Med.* **1979**, *8*, 249–265. [CrossRef]
50. Greenwald, R.A.; Kirkwood, K. Adult periodontitis as a model for rheumatoid arthritis (with emphasis on treatment strategies). *J. Rheumatol.* **1999**, *26*, 1650–1653.
51. Katz, J.; Goultschin, J.; Benoliel, R.; Brautbar, C. Human leukocyte antigen (HLA) DR4. Positive association with rapidly progressing periodontitis. *J. Periodontol.* **1987**, *58*, 607–610. [CrossRef]
52. Bonfil, J.J.; Dillier, F.L.; Mercier, P.; Reviron, D.; Foti, B.; Sambuc, R.; Brodeur, J.M.; Sedarat, C. A "case control" study on the role of HLA DR4 in severe periodontitis and rapidly progressive periodontitis. Identification of types and subtypes using molecular biology (PCR.SSO). *J. Clin. Periodontol.* **1999**, *26*, 77–84. [CrossRef]
53. Rizzo, A.A.; Mitchell, C.T. Chronic allergic inflammation induced by repeated deposition of antigen in rabbit gingival pockets. *Periodontics* **1966**, *4*, 5.
54. McHugh, W.D. Some aspects of the development of gingival epithelium. *Periodontics* **1963**, *1*, 239–244.

55. Schroeder, H. Quantitative parameters of early human gingival inflammation. *Arch. Oral Biol.* **1970**, *15*, 383–IN4. [CrossRef]
56. Sugawara, M.; Yamashita, K.; Yoshie, H.; Hara, K. Detection of, and anti-collagen antibody produced by, CD5-positive B cells in inflamed gingival tissues. *J. Periodontal Res.* **1992**, *27*, 489–498. [CrossRef]
57. Kristoffersen, T.; Tonder, O. Anti-immunoglobulin activity in inflamed human gingiva. *J. Dent. Res.* **1973**, *52*, 991.
58. Gargiulo, A.V.; Robinson, J.; Toto, P.D.; Gargiulo, A.W. Identification of Rheumatoid Factor in Periodontal Disease. *J. Periodontol.* **1982**, *53*, 568–577. [CrossRef]
59. Gargiulo, A.V., Jr.; Toto, P.D.; Robinson, J.A.; Gargiulo, A.W. Latex slide agglutination vs. ELISA system: Rheumatoid factor detection in inflamed human gingiva. *J. Periodontal Res.* **1985**, *20*, 31–34. [CrossRef]
60. Malmström, M.; Natvig, J.B. IgG Rheumatoid Factor in Dental Periapical Lesions of Patients with Rheumatoid Disease. *Scand. J. Rheumatol.* **1975**, *4*, 177–185. [CrossRef]
61. McGraw, W.T.; Potempa, J.; Farley, D.; Travis, J. Purification, Characterization, and Sequence Analysis of a Potential Virulence Factor from Porphyromonas gingivalis, Peptidylarginine Deiminase. *Infect. Immun.* **1999**, *67*, 3248–3256.
62. Rosenstein, E.D.; Greenwald, R.A.; Kushner, L.J.; Weissmann, G. Hypothesis: The Humoral Immune Response to Oral Bacteria Provides a Stimulus for the Development of Rheumatoid Arthritis. *Inflammation* **2004**, *28*, 311–318. [CrossRef]
63. Schellekens, G.A.; De Jong, B.A.; Hoogen, F.H.V.D.; Van De Putte, L.B.; Van Venrooij, W.J. Citrulline is an essential constituent of antigenic determinants recognized by rheumatoid arthritis-specific autoantibodies. *J. Clin. Investig.* **1998**, *101*, 273–281. [CrossRef]
64. Kaur, S.; White, S.; Bartold, P.M. Periodontal disease and rheumatoid arthritis: A systematic review. *J. Dent. Res.* **2013**, *92*, 399–408. [CrossRef]
65. Fuggle, N.R.; Smith, T.O.; Kaul, A.; Sofat, N. Hand to Mouth: A Systematic Review and Meta-Analysis of the Association between Rheumatoid Arthritis and Periodontitis. *Front. Immunol.* **2016**, *7*, 80. [CrossRef]
66. Araujo, V.M.; Melo, I.M.; Lima, V. Relationship between Periodontitis and Rheumatoid Arthritis: Review of the Literature. *Med.iat. Inflamm.* **2015**, *2015*, 259074. [CrossRef]
67. Kindstedt, E.; Johansson, L.; Palmqvist, P.; Holm, C.K.; Kokkonen, H.; Johansson, I.; Dahlqvist, S.R.; Lundberg, P. Association Between Marginal Jawbone Loss and Onset of Rheumatoid Arthritis and Relationship to Plasma Levels of RANKL. *Arthritis Rheumatol.* **2018**, *70*, 508–515. [CrossRef]
68. Eriksson, K.; Nise, L.; Kats, A.; Luttropp, E.; Catrina, A.I.; Askling, J.; Jansson, L.; Alfredsson, L.; Klareskog, L.; Lundberg, K.; et al. Prevalence of Periodontitis in Patients with Established Rheumatoid Arthritis: A Swedish Population Based Case-Control Study. *PLoS ONE* **2016**, *11*, e0155956. [CrossRef]
69. Sjöström, L.; Laurell, L.; Hugoson, A.; Håkansson, J.P. Periodontal conditions in adults with rheumatoid arthritis. *Community Dent. Oral Epidemiol.* **1989**, *17*, 234–236. [CrossRef]
70. Eke, P.I.; Dye, B.A.; Wei, L.; Thornton-Evans, G.O.; Genco, R.J. CDC Periodontal Disease Surveillance workgroup: James Beck GDRP. Prevalence of periodontitis in adults in the United States: 2009 and 2010. *J. Dent. Res.* **2012**, *91*, 914–920. [CrossRef]
71. Kassebaum, N.J.; Bernabe, E.; Dahiya, M.; Bhandari, B.; Murray, C.J.; Marcenes, W. Global burden of severe periodontitis in 1990-2010, a systematic review and meta-regression. *J. Dent. Res.* **2014**, *93*, 1045–1053. [CrossRef]
72. dos Anjos, L.M.; Pereira, I.A.; 'Orsi, E.; Seaman, A.P.; Burlingame, R.W.; Morato, E.F. A comparative study of IgG second- and third-generation anti-cyclic citrullinated peptide (CCP) ELISAs and their combination with IgA third-generation CCP ELISA for the diagnosis of rheumatoid arthritis. *Clin. Rheumatol.* **2009**, *28*, 153–158. [CrossRef]
73. Lutteri, L.; Malaise, M.; Chapelle, J.P. Comparison of second- and third-generation anti-cyclic citrullinated peptide antibodies assays for detecting rheumatoid arthritis. *Clin. Chim. Acta* **2007**, *386*, 76–81. [CrossRef]
74. Sugawara, K.; Fujisaki, M. Properties of Peptidylarginine Deiminase from the Epidermis of Newborn Rats. *J. Biochem.* **1981**, *89*, 257–263.
75. Raijmakers, R.; Zendman, A.J.; Egberts, W.V.; Vossenaar, E.R.; Raats, J.; Soede-Huijbregts, C.; Rutjes, F.P.; Van Veelen, P.A.; Drijfhout, J.W.; Pruijn, G.J. Methylation of Arginine Residues Interferes with Citrullination by Peptidylarginine Deiminases in vitro. *J. Mol. Biol.* **2007**, *367*, 1118–1129. [CrossRef]

76. Kinloch, A.; Lundberg, K.; Wait, R.; Wegner, N.; Lim, N.H.; Zendman, A.J.W.; Saxne, T.; Malmstr, V.; Venables, P.J.; Kinloch, A. Synovial fluid is a site of citrullination of autoantigens in inflammatory arthritis. *Arthritis Rheum.* **2008**, *58*, 2287–2295. [CrossRef]
77. Foulquier, C.; Sebbag, M.; Clavel, C.; Chapuy-Regaud, S.; Al Badine, R.; Méchin, M.C.; Vincent, C.; Nachat, R.; Yamada, M.; Takahara, H.; et al. Peptidyl arginine deiminase type 2 (PAD-2) and PAD-4 but not PAD-1, PAD-3, and PAD-6 are expressed in rheumatoid arthritis synovium in close association with tissue inflammation. *Arthritis Rheum.* **2007**, *56*, 3541–3553. [CrossRef]
78. Chang, X.; Yamada, R.; Suzuki, A.; Sawada, T.; Yoshino, S.; Tokuhiro, S.; Yamamoto, K. Localization of peptidylarginine deiminase 4 (PADI4) and citrullinated protein in synovial tissue of rheumatoid arthritis. *Rheumatology (Oxf.)* **2005**, *44*, 40–50. [CrossRef]
79. Arita, K.; Hashimoto, H.; Shimizu, T.; Nakashima, K.; Yamada, M.; Sato, M. Structural basis for Ca^{2+}-induced activation of human PAD4. *Nat. Struct. Mol. Biol.* **2004**, *11*, 777–783. [CrossRef]
80. Slade, D.J.; Fang, P.; Dreyton, C.J.; Zhang, Y.; Fuhrmann, J.; Rempel, D.; Bax, B.D.; Coonrod, S.A.; Lewis, H.D.; Guo, M.; et al. Protein Arginine Deiminase 2 Binds Calcium in an Ordered Fashion: Implications for Inhibitor Design. *ACS Chem. Biol.* **2015**, *10*, 1043–1053. [CrossRef]
81. Saijo, S.; Nagai, A.; Kinjo, S.; Mashimo, R.; Akimoto, M.; Kizawa, K.; Yabe-Wada, T.; Shimizu, N.; Takahara, H.; Unno, M. Monomeric Form of Peptidylarginine Deiminase Type I Revealed by X-ray Crystallography and Small-Angle X-ray Scattering. *J. Mol. Biol.* **2016**, *428*, 3058–3073. [CrossRef]
82. Kearney, P.L.; Bhatia, M.; Jones, N.G.; Yuan, L.; Glascock, M.C.; Catchings, K.L.; Yamada, M.; Thompson, P.R. Kinetic Characterization of Protein Arginine Deiminase 4: A Transcriptional Corepressor Implicated in the Onset and Progression of Rheumatoid Arthritis. *Biochemistry* **2005**, *44*, 10570–10582. [CrossRef]
83. Vossenaar, E.R.; Zendman, A.J.; Van Venrooij, W.J.; Pruijn, G.J. PAD, a growing family of citrullinating enzymes: Genes, features and involvement in disease. *BioEssays* **2003**, *25*, 1106–1118. [CrossRef]
84. Witalison, E.E.; Thompson, P.R.; Hofseth, L.J. Protein Arginine Deiminases and Associated Citrullination: Physiological Functions and Diseases Associated with Dysregulation. *Curr. Drug Targets* **2015**, *16*, 700–710. [CrossRef]
85. Lee, C.Y.; Wang, D.; Wilhelm, M.; Zolg, D.P.; Schmidt, T.; Schnatbaum, K.; Reimer, U.; Ponten, F.; Uhlen, M.; Hahne, H.; et al. Mining the Human Tissue Proteome for Protein Citrullination. *Mol. Cell. Proteom.* **2018**, *17*, 1378–1391. [CrossRef]
86. van Beers, J.J.; Schwarte, C.M.; Stammen-Vogelzangs, J.; Oosterink, E.; Bozic, B.; Pruijn, G.J. The rheumatoid arthritis synovial fluid citrullinome reveals novel citrullinated epitopes in apolipoprotein E, myeloid nuclear differentiation antigen, and beta-actin. *Arthritis Rheum.* **2013**, *65*, 69–80. [CrossRef]
87. Romero, V.; Fert-Bober, J.; Nigrovic, P.A.; Darrah, E.; Haque, U.J.; Lee, D.M.; Van Eyk, J.; Rosen, A.; Andrade, F. Immune-Mediated Pore-Forming Pathways Induce Cellular Hypercitrullination and Generate Citrullinated Autoantigens in Rheumatoid Arthritis. *Sci. Transl. Med.* **2013**, *5*, 209ra150. [CrossRef]
88. Tutturen, A.E.V.; Fleckenstein, B.; De Souza, G.A. Assessing the Citrullinome in Rheumatoid Arthritis Synovial Fluid with and without Enrichment of Citrullinated Peptides. *J. Proteome Res.* **2014**, *13*, 2867–2873. [CrossRef]
89. Wang, F.; Chen, F.F.; Gao, W.B.; Wang, H.Y.; Zhao, N.W.; Xu, M.; Gao, D.Y.; Yu, W.; Yan, X.L.; Zhao, J.N.; et al. Identification of citrullinated peptides in the synovial fluid of patients with rheumatoid arthritis using LC-MALDI-TOF/TOF. *Clin. Rheumatol.* **2016**, *35*, 2185–2194. [CrossRef]
90. Tilvawala, R.; Nguyen, S.H.; Maurais, A.J.; Nemmara, V.V.; Nagar, M.; Salinger, A.J.; Nagpal, S.; Weerapana, E.; Thompson, P.R. The Rheumatoid Arthritis-Associated Citrullinome. *Cell Chem. Biol.* **2018**, *25*, 691–704.e6. [CrossRef]
91. Bennike, T.B.; Ellingsen, T.; Glerup, H.; Bonderup, O.K.; Carlsen, T.G.; Meyer, M.K.; Bøgsted, M.; Christiansen, G.; Birkelund, S.; Andersen, V.; et al. Proteome Analysis of Rheumatoid Arthritis Gut Mucosa. *J. Proteome Res.* **2017**, *16*, 346–354. [CrossRef]
92. Konig, M.F.; Abusleme, L.; Reinholdt, J.; Palmer, R.J.; Teles, R.P.; Sampson, K.; Rosen, A.; Nigrovic, P.A.; Sokolove, J.; Giles, J.T.; et al. Aggregatibacter actinomycetemcomitans-induced hypercitrullination links periodontal infection to autoimmunity in rheumatoid arthritis. *Sci. Transl. Med.* **2016**, *8*, 369ra176. [CrossRef]
93. Schwenzer, A.; Quirke, A.M.; Marzeda, A.M.; Wong, A.; Montgomery, A.B.; Sayles, H.R.; Eick, S.; Gawron, K.; Chomyszyn-Gajewska, M.; et al. Association of Distinct Fine Specificities of Anti-Citrullinated Peptide

Antibodies with Elevated Immune Responses to Prevotella intermedia in a Subgroup of Patients With Rheumatoid Arthritis and Periodontitis. *Arthritis Rheumatol.* **2017**, *69*, 2303–2313. [CrossRef]

94. Macdonald, J.B.; Gibbons, R.J.; Socransky, S.S. Bacterial mechanisms in periodontal disease. *Ann. N. Y. Acad. Sci.* **1960**, *85*, 467–478. [CrossRef]
95. Finegold, S.M.; Barnes, E.M. Report of Icsb Taxonomic Subcommittee on Gram-Negative Anaerobic Rods. *Int. J. Syst. Bacteriol.* **1977**, *27*, 388–391. [CrossRef]
96. Reed, M.J.; Slots, J.; Mouton, C.; Genco, R.J. Antigenic Studies of Oral and Non-Oral Black-Pigmented Bacteroides Strains. *Infect. Immun.* **1980**, *29*, 564–574.
97. Kaczmarek, F.S.; Coykendall, A.L. Production of phenylacetic acid by strains of *Bacteroides asaccharolyticus* and *Bacteroides gingivalis* (sp. nov). *J. Clin. Microbiol.* **1980**, *12*, 288–290.
98. Shah, H.N.; Collins, M.D. Proposal for Reclassification of Bacteroides asaccharolyticus, Bacteroides gingivalis, and Bacteroides endodontalis in a New Genus, Porphyromonas. *Int. J. Syst. Bacteriol.* **1988**, *38*, 128–131. [CrossRef]
99. Lamont, R.J.; Koo, H.; Hajishengallis, G. The oral microbiota: Dynamic communities and host interactions. *Nat. Rev. Genet.* **2018**, *16*, 745–759. [CrossRef]
100. Hajishengallis, G.; Darveau, R.P.; Curtis, M.A. The keystone-pathogen hypothesis. *Nat. Rev. Microbiol.* **2012**, *10*, 717–725. [CrossRef]
101. de Smit, M.; Westra, J.; Vissink, A.; Doornbos-van der Meer, B.; Brouwer, E.; van Winkelhoff, A.J. Periodontitis in established rheumatoid arthritis patients: A cross-sectional clinical, microbiological and serological study. *Arthritis Res. Ther.* **2012**, *14*, R222. [CrossRef]
102. Engström, M.; Eriksson, K.; Lee, L.; Hermansson, M.; Johansson, A.; Nicholas, A.P.; Gerasimcik, N.; Lundberg, K.; Klareskog, L.; Catrina, A.I.; et al. Increased citrullination and expression of peptidylarginine deiminases independently of *P. gingivalis* and *A. actinomycetemcomitans* in gingival tissue of patients with periodontitis. *J. Transl. Med.* **2018**, *16*, 214. [CrossRef]
103. Eriksson, K.; Fei, G.; Lundmark, A.; Benchimol, D.; Lee, L.; Hu, Y.O.O.; Kats, A.; Saevarsdottir, S.; Catrina, A.I.; Klinge, B.; et al. Periodontal Health and Oral Microbiota in Patients with Rheumatoid Arthritis. *J. Clin. Med.* **2019**, *8*, 630. [CrossRef]
104. Schmickler, J.; Rupprecht, A.; Patschan, S.; Patschan, D.; Müller, G.A.; Haak, R.; Mausberg, R.F.; Schmalz, G.; Kottmann, T.; Ziebolz, D.; et al. Cross-Sectional Evaluation of Periodontal Status and Microbiologic and Rheumatoid Parameters in a Large Cohort of Patients with Rheumatoid Arthritis. *J. Periodontol.* **2017**, *88*, 368–379. [CrossRef]
105. Ziebolz, D.; Pabel, S.O.; Lange, K.; Krohn-Grimberghe, B.; Hornecker, E.; Mausberg, R.F. Clinical Periodontal and Microbiologic Parameters in Patients with Rheumatoid Arthritis. *J. Periodontol.* **2011**, *82*, 1424–1432. [CrossRef]
106. Beyer, K.; Zaura, E.; Brandt, B.W.; Buijs, M.J.; Brun, J.G.; Crielaard, W.; Bolstad, A.I. Subgingival microbiome of rheumatoid arthritis patients in relation to their disease status and periodontal health. *PLoS ONE* **2018**, *13*, e0202278. [CrossRef]
107. Laugisch, O.; Wong, A.; Sroka, A.; Kantyka, T.; Koziel, J.; Neuhaus, K.; Sculean, A.; Venables, P.J.; Potempa, J.; Möller, B.; et al. Citrullination in the periodontium—A possible link between periodontitis and rheumatoid arthritis. *Clin. Oral Investig.* **2015**, *20*, 675–683. [CrossRef]
108. Lopez-Oliva, I.; Paropkari, A.D.; Saraswat, S.; Serban, S.; Yonel, Z.; Sharma, P.; De Pablo, P.; Raza, K.; Filer, A.; Chapple, I.; et al. Dysbiotic Subgingival Microbial Communities in Periodontally Healthy Patients with Rheumatoid Arthritis. *Arthritis Rheumatol.* **2018**, *70*, 1008–1013. [CrossRef]
109. Zhang, X.; Zhang, D.; Jia, H.; Feng, Q.; Wang, D.; Liang, D.; Wu, X.; Li, J.; Tang, L.; Li, Y.; et al. The oral and gut microbiomes are perturbed in rheumatoid arthritis and partly normalized after treatment. *Nat. Med.* **2015**, *21*, 895–905. [CrossRef]
110. Mikuls, T.R.; Walker, C.; Qiu, F.; Yu, F.; Thiele, G.M.; Alfant, B.; Li, E.C.; Zhao, L.Y.; Wang, G.P.; Datta, S.; et al. The subgingival microbiome in patients with established rheumatoid arthritis. *Rheumatology* **2018**, *57*, 1162–1172. [CrossRef]
111. Scher, J.U.; Ubeda, C.; Equinda, M.; Khanin, R.; Buischi, Y.; Viale, A.; Lipuma, L.; Attur, M.; Pillinger, M.H.; Weissmann, G.; et al. Periodontal Disease and the Oral Microbiota in New-Onset Rheumatoid Arthritis. *Arthritis Rheum.* **2012**, *64*, 3083–3094. [CrossRef]

112. Mankia, K.; Cheng, Z.; Do, T.; Hunt, L.; Meade, J.; Kang, J.; Clerehugh, V.; Speirs, A.; Tugnait, A.; Hensor, E.M.A.; et al. Prevalence of Periodontal Disease and Periodontopathic Bacteria in Anti–Cyclic Citrullinated Protein Antibody–Positive At-Risk Adults Without Arthritis. *JAMA Netw. Open* **2019**, *2*, e195394. [CrossRef]
113. Arvikar, S.L.; Collier, D.S.; Fisher, M.C.; Unizony, S.; Cohen, G.L.; McHugh, G.; Kawai, T.; Strle, K.; Steere, A.C. Clinical correlations with Porphyromonas gingivalis antibody responses in patients with early rheumatoid arthritis. *Arthritis Res. Ther.* **2013**, *15*, R109. [CrossRef]
114. Okada, M.; Kobayashi, T.; Ito, S.; Yokoyama, T.; Komatsu, Y.; Abe, A.; Murasawa, A.; Yoshie, H. Antibody Responses to Periodontopathic Bacteria in Relation to Rheumatoid Arthritis in Japanese Adults. *J. Periodontol.* **2011**, *82*, 1433–1441. [CrossRef]
115. Mikuls, T.R.; Payne, J.B.; Reinhardt, R.A.; Thiele, G.M.; Maziarz, E.; Cannella, A.C.; Holers, V.M.; Kuhn, K.A.; O'Dell, J.R. Antibody responses to Porphyromonas gingivalis (P. gingivalis) in subjects with rheumatoid arthritis and periodontitis. *Int. Immunopharmacol.* **2009**, *9*, 38–42. [CrossRef]
116. Ogrendik, M.; Kokino, S.; Ozdemir, F.; Bird, P.S.; Hamlet, S. Serum Antibodies to Oral Anaerobic Bacteria in Patients with Rheumatoid Arthritis. *MedGenMed Medscape Gen. Med.* **2005**, *7*, 2.
117. Yusof, Z.R.; Porter, S.; Greenman, J.; Scully, C. Levels of Serum IgG against Porphyromonas gingivalis in Patients with Rapidly Progressive Periodontitis, Rheumatoid Arthritis and Adult Periodontitis. *J. Nihon Univ. Sch. Dent.* **1995**, *37*, 197–200. [CrossRef]
118. Moen, K.; Brun, J.G.; Madland, T.M.; Tynning, T.; Jonsson, R. Immunoglobulin G and a Antibody Responses to Bacteroides forsythus and Prevotella intermedia in Sera and Synovial Fluids of Arthritis Patients. *Clin. Diagn. Lab. Immunol.* **2003**, *10*, 1043–1050. [CrossRef]
119. de Smit, M.; van de Stadt, L.A.; Janssen, K.M.; Doornbos-van der Meer, B.; Vissink, A.; van Winkelhoff, A.J.; Brouwer, E.; Westra, J.; van Schaardenburg, D. Antibodies against Porphyromonas gingivalis in seropositive arthralgia patients do not predict development of rheumatoid arthritis. *Ann. Rheum. Dis.* **2014**, *73*, 1277–1279. [CrossRef]
120. Konig, M.F.; Paracha, A.S.; Moni, M.; Bingham, C.O., III; Andrade, F. Defining the role of Porphyromonas gingivalis peptidylarginine deiminase (PPAD) in rheumatoid arthritis through the study of PPAD biology. *Ann. Rheum. Dis.* **2015**, *74*, 2054–2061. [CrossRef]
121. Quirke, A.M.; Lugli, E.B.; Wegner, N.; Hamilton, B.C.; Charles, P.; Chowdhury, M.; Ytterberg, A.J.; Zubarev, R.A.; Potempa, J.; Culshaw, S.; et al. Heightened immune response to autocitrullinated Porphyromonas gingivalis peptidylarginine deiminase: A potential mechanism for breaching immunologic tolerance in rheumatoid arthritis. *Ann. Rheum. Dis.* **2014**, *73*, 263–269. [CrossRef]
122. Fisher, B.A.; Cartwright, A.J.; Quirke, A.M.; de Pablo, P.; Romaguera, D.; Panico, S.; Mattiello, A.; Gavrila, D.; Navarro, C.; Sacerdote, C.; et al. Smoking, Porphyromonas gingivalis and the immune response to citrullinated autoantigens before the clinical onset of rheumatoid arthritis in a Southern European nested case-control study. *BMC Musculoskelet. Disord.* **2015**, *16*, 331. [CrossRef]
123. Johansson, L.; Sherina, N.; Kharlamova, N.; Potempa, B.; Larsson, B.; Israelsson, L.; Potempa, J.; Rantapää-Dahlqvist, S.; Lundberg, K. Concentration of antibodies against Porphyromonas gingivalis is increased before the onset of symptoms of rheumatoid arthritis. *Arthritis Res. Ther.* **2016**, *18*, 201. [CrossRef]
124. Kharlamova, N.; Jiang, X.; Sherina, N.; Potempa, B.; Israelsson, L.; Quirke, A.-M.; Eriksson, K.; Yucel-Lindberg, T.; Venables, P.J.; Potempa, J.; et al. Antibodies to Porphyromonas gingivalis indicate interaction between oral infection, smoking and risk genes in rheumatoid arthritis etiology. *Arthritis Rheumatol.* **2016**, *68*, 604–613. [CrossRef]
125. Mikuls, T.R.; Payne, J.B.; Yu, F.; Thiele, G.M.; Reynolds, R.J.; Cannon, G.W.; Markt, J.; McGowan, D.; Kerr, G.S.; Redman, R.S.; et al. Periodontitis and Porphyromonas gingivalis in Patients with Rheumatoid Arthritis. *Arthritis Rheumatol.* **2014**, *66*, 1090–1100. [CrossRef]
126. Okada, M.; Kobayashi, T.; Ito, S.; Yokoyama, T.; Abe, A.; Murasawa, A.; Yoshie, H. Periodontal Treatment Decreases Levels of Antibodies to Porphyromonas gingivalis and Citrulline in Patients with Rheumatoid Arthritis and Periodontitis. *J. Periodontol.* **2013**, *84*, e74–e84. [CrossRef]
127. Rinaudo-Gaujous, M.; Blasco-Baque, V.; Miossec, P.; Gaudin, P.; Farge, P.; Roblin, X.; Thomas, T.; Paul, S.; Marotte, H. Infliximab Induced a Dissociated Response of Severe Periodontal Biomarkers in Rheumatoid Arthritis Patients. *J. Clin. Med.* **2019**, *8*, 751. [CrossRef]

128. Stobernack, T.; Glasner, C.; Junker, S.; Gabarrini, G.; De Smit, M.; Van Winkelhoff, A.J.; De Jong, A.; Otto, A.; Becher, D.; Van Dijl, J.M. Extracellular Proteome and Citrullinome of the Oral Pathogen Porphyromonas gingivalis. *J. Proteome Res.* **2016**, *15*, 4532–4543. [CrossRef]
129. Bae, S.C.; Lee, Y.H. Association between anti-Porphyromonas gingivalis antibody, anti-citrullinated protein antibodies, and rheumatoid arthritis a meta-analysis. *Z. Für Rheumatol.* **2018**, *77*, 522–532. [CrossRef]
130. Bender, P.; Burgin, W.B.; Sculean, A.; Eick, S. Serum antibody levels against Porphyromonas gingivalis in patients with and without rheumatoid arthritis - a systematic review and meta-analysis. *Clin. Oral Investig.* **2017**, *21*, 33–42. [CrossRef]
131. Maresz, K.J.; Hellvard, A.; Sroka, A.; Adamowicz, K.; Bielecka, E.; Koziel, J.; Gawron, K.; Mizgalska, D.; Marcinska, K.A.; Benedyk, M.; et al. Porphyromonas gingivalis Facilitates the Development and Progression of Destructive Arthritis through Its Unique Bacterial Peptidylarginine Deiminase (PAD). *PLoS Pathog.* **2013**, *9*, e1003627. [CrossRef]
132. de Aquino, S.G.; Abdollahi-Roodsaz, S.; Koenders, M.I.; van de Loo, F.A.; Pruijn, G.J.; Marijnissen, R.J.; Walgreen, B.; Helsen, M.M.; van den Bersselaar, L.A.; de Molon, R.S.; et al. Periodontal pathogens directly promote autoimmune experimental arthritis by inducing a TLR2- and IL-1-driven Th17 response. *J. Immunol.* **2014**, *192*, 4103–4111. [CrossRef]
133. de Aquino, S.G.; Talbot, J.; Sônego, F.; Turato, W.M.; Grespan, R.; Avila-Campos, M.J.; Cunha, F.Q.; Cirelli, J.A. The aggravation of arthritis by periodontitis is dependent of IL-17 receptor a activation. *J. Clin. Periodontol.* **2017**, *44*, 881–891. [CrossRef]
134. Marchesan, J.T.; Gerow, E.A.; Schaff, R.; Taut, A.D.; Shin, S.Y.; Sugai, J.; Brand, D.; Burberry, A.; Jorns, J.; Lundy, S.K.; et al. Porphyromonas gingivalis oral infection exacerbates the development and severity of collagen-induced arthritis. *Arthritis Res. Ther.* **2013**, *15*, R186. [CrossRef]
135. Jung, H.; Jung, S.M.; Rim, Y.A.; Park, N.; Nam, Y.; Lee, J.; Park, S.H.; Ju, J.H. Arthritic role of Porphyromonas gingivalis in collagen-induced arthritis mice. *PLoS ONE* **2017**, *12*, e0188698. [CrossRef]
136. Chukkapalli, S.; Rivera-Kweh, M.; Gehlot, P.; Velsko, I.; Bhattacharyya, I.; Calise, S.J.; Satoh, M.; Chan, E.K.L.; Holoshitz, J.; Kesavalu, L. Periodontal bacterial colonization in synovial tissues exacerbates collagen-induced arthritis in B10.RIII mice. *Arthritis Res. Ther.* **2016**, *18*, 161. [CrossRef]
137. Sato, K.; Takahashi, N.; Kato, T.; Matsuda, Y.; Yokoji, M.; Yamada, M.; Nakajima, T.; Kondo, N.; Endo, N.; Yamamoto, R.; et al. Aggravation of collagen-induced arthritis by orally administered Porphyromonas gingivalis through modulation of the gut microbiota and gut immune system. *Sci. Rep.* **2017**, *7*, 6955. [CrossRef]
138. Yamakawa, M.; Ouhara, K.; Kajiya, M.; Munenaga, S.; Kittaka, M.; Yamasaki, S.; Takeda, K.; Takeshita, K.; Mizuno, N.; Fujita, T.; et al. Porphyromonas gingivalis infection exacerbates the onset of rheumatoid arthritis in SKG mice. *Clin. Exp. Immunol.* **2016**, *186*, 177–189. [CrossRef]
139. Sandal, I.; Karydis, A.; Luo, J.; Prislovsky, A.; Whittington, K.B.; Rosloniec, E.F.; Dong, C.; Novack, D.V.; Mydel, P.; Zheng, S.G.; et al. Bone loss and aggravated autoimmune arthritis in HLA-DR beta 1-bearing humanized mice following oral challenge with Porphyromonas gingivalis. *Arthritis Res. Ther.* **2016**, *18*, 249. [CrossRef]
140. Gully, N.; Bright, R.; Marino, V.; Marchant, C.; Cantley, M.; Haynes, D.; Butler, C.; Dashper, S.; Reynolds, E.; Bartold, M. Porphyromonas gingivalis Peptidylarginine Deiminase, a Key Contributor in the Pathogenesis of Experimental Periodontal Disease and Experimental Arthritis. *PLoS ONE* **2014**, *9*, e100838. [CrossRef]
141. Munenaga, S.; Ouhara, K.; Hamamoto, Y.; Kajiya, M.; Takeda, K.; Yamasaki, S.; Kawai, T.; Mizuno, N.; Fujita, T.; Sugiyama, E.; et al. The involvement of C5a in the progression of experimental arthritis with Porphyromonas gingivalis infection in SKG mice. *Arthritis Res. Ther.* **2018**, *20*, 247. [CrossRef]
142. Ebbers, M.; Lübcke, P.M.; Volzke, J.; Kriebel, K.; Hieke, C.; Engelmann, R.; Lang, H.; Kreikemeyer, B.; Müller-Hilke, B.; et al. Interplay between P. gingivalis, F. nucleatum and A. actinomycetemcomitans in murine alveolar bone loss, arthritis onset and progression. *Sci. Rep.* **2018**, *8*, 15129. [CrossRef]
143. Eriksson, K.; Lönnblom, E.; Tour, G.; Kats, A.; Mydel, P.; Georgsson, P.; Hultgren, C.; Kharlamova, N.; Norin, U.; Jönsson, J.; et al. Effects by periodontitis on pristane-induced arthritis in rats. *J. Transl. Med.* **2016**, *14*, 311. [CrossRef]
144. Courbon, G.; Rinaudo-Gaujous, M.; Blasco-Baque, V.; Auger, I.; Caire, R.; Mijola, L.; Vico, L.; Paul, S.; Marotte, H. Porphyromonas gingivalis experimentally induces periodontis and an anti-CCP2-associated arthritis in the rat. *Ann. Rheum. Dis.* **2019**, *78*, 594–599. [CrossRef]

145. Kinloch, A.J.; Alzabin, S.; Brintnell, W.; Wilson, E.; Barra, L.; Wegner, N.; Bell, D.A.; Cairns, E.; Venables, P.J. Immunization with Porphyromonas gingivalis enolase induces autoimmunity to mammalian alpha-enolase and arthritis in DR4-IE-transgenic mice. *Arthritis Rheum.* **2011**, *63*, 3818–3823. [CrossRef]
146. Mangat, P.; Wegner, N.; Venables, P.J.; Potempa, J. Bacterial and human peptidylarginine deiminases: Targets for inhibiting the autoimmune response in rheumatoid arthritis? *Arthritis Res. Ther.* **2010**, *12*, 209. [CrossRef]
147. Hayashi, H.; Morioka, M.; Ichimiya, S.; Yamato, K.; Hinode, D.; Nagata, A.; Nakamura, R. Participation of an arginyl residue of insulin chain B in the inhibition of hemagglutination by Porphyromonas gingivalis. *Oral Microbiol. Immunol.* **1993**, *8*, 386–389. [CrossRef]
148. Goulas, T.; Mizgalska, D.; Garcia-Ferrer, I.; Kantyka, T.; Guevara, T.; Szmigielski, B.; Sroka, A.; Millán, C.; Usón, I.; Veillard, F.; et al. Structure and mechanism of a bacterial host-protein citrullinating virulence factor, Porphyromonas gingivalis peptidylarginine deiminase. *Sci. Rep.* **2015**, *5*, 11969. [CrossRef]
149. Montgomery, A.B.; Kopec, J.; Shrestha, L.; Thezenas, M.L.; Burgess-Brown, N.A.; Fischer, R.; Yue, W.W.; Venables, P.J. Crystal structure of Porphyromonas gingivalis peptidylarginine deiminase: Implications for autoimmunity in rheumatoid arthritis. *Ann. Rheum. Dis.* **2016**, *75*, 1255–1261. [CrossRef]
150. Bereta, G.; Goulas, T.; Madej, M.; Bielecka, E.; Solà, M.; Potempa, J.; Gomis-Rüth, F.X. Structure, function, and inhibition of a genomic/clinical variant of Porphyromonas gingivalis peptidylarginine deiminase. *Protein Sci.* **2019**, *28*, 478–486. [CrossRef]
151. Gabarrini, G.; Heida, R.; Van Ieperen, N.; Curtis, M.A.; Van Winkelhoff, A.J.; Van Dijl, J.M. Dropping anchor: Attachment of peptidylarginine deiminase via A-LPS to secreted outer membrane vesicles of Porphyromonas gingivalis. *Sci. Rep.* **2018**, *8*, 8949. [CrossRef]
152. Gabarrini, G.; Medina, L.M.P.; Stobernack, T.; Prins, R.C.; Espina, M.D.T.; Kuipers, J.; Chlebowicz, M.A.; Rossen, J.W.A.; Van Winkelhoff, A.J.; Van Dijl, J.M. There's no place like OM: Vesicular sorting and secretion of the peptidylarginine deiminase of Porphyromonas gingivalis. *Virulence* **2018**, *9*, 456–464. [CrossRef]
153. Casiano-Colón, A.; Marquis, R.E. Role of the arginine deiminase system in protecting oral bacteria and an enzymatic basis for acid tolerance. *Appl. Environ. Microbiol.* **1988**, *54*, 1318–1324.
154. Niederman, R.; Brunkhorst, B.; Smith, S.; Weinreb, R.; Ryder, M. Ammonia as a potential mediator of adult human periodontal infection: Inhibition of neutrophil function. *Arch. Oral Biol.* **1990**, *35*, S205–S209. [CrossRef]
155. Shawcross, D.L.; Wright, G.A.K.; Stadlbauer, V.; Hodges, S.J.; Davies, N.A.; Wheeler-Jones, C.; Pitsillides, A.A.; Jalan, R. Ammonia impairs neutrophil phagocytic function in liver disease. *Hepatology* **2008**, *48*, 1202–1212. [CrossRef]
156. Wegner, N.; Wait, R.; Sroka, A.; Eick, S.; Nguyen, K.A.; Lundberg, K.; Kinloch, A.; Culshaw, S.; Potempa, J.; Venables, P.J. Peptidylarginine deiminase from Porphyromonas gingivalis citrullinates human fibrinogen and alpha-enolase: Implications for autoimmunity in rheumatoid arthritis. *Arthritis Rheum.* **2010**, *62*, 2662–2672. [CrossRef]
157. Li, S.; Yu, Y.; Yue, Y.; Liao, H.; Xie, W.; Thai, J.; Mikuls, T.R.; Thiele, G.M.; Duryee, M.J.; Sayles, H.; et al. Autoantibodies from Single Circulating Plasmablasts React With Citrullinated Antigens and Porphyromonas gingivalis in Rheumatoid Arthritis. *Arthritis Rheumatol.* **2016**, *68*, 614–626. [CrossRef]
158. Rodríguez, S.B.; Stitt, B.L.; Ash, D.E. Expression of Peptidylarginine Deiminase from Porphyromonas gingivalis in Escherichia coli: Enzyme Purification and Characterization. *Arch. Biochem. Biophys.* **2009**, *488*, 14–22. [CrossRef]
159. Sato, K.; Yukitake, H.; Narita, Y.; Shoji, M.; Naito, M.; Nakayama, K. Identification of Porphyromonas gingivalis proteins secreted by the Por secretion system. *FEMS Microbiol. Lett.* **2013**, *338*, 68–76. [CrossRef]
160. Shoji, M.; Sato, K.; Yukitake, H.; Kondo, Y.; Narita, Y.; Kadowaki, T.; Naito, M.; Nakayama, K. Por Secretion System-Dependent Secretion and Glycosylation of Porphyromonas gingivalis Hemin-Binding Protein 35. *PLoS ONE* **2011**, *6*, e21372. [CrossRef]
161. Konig, M.F.; Bingham, C.O., III; Andrade, F. PPAD is not targeted as a citrullinated protein in rheumatoid arthritis, but remains a candidate for inducing autoimmunity. *Ann. Rheum. Dis.* **2015**, *74*, e8. [CrossRef]
162. Quirke, A.-M.; Lundberg, K.; Potempa, J.; Mikuls, T.R.; Venables, P.J. PPAD remains a credible candidate for inducing autoimmunity in rheumatoid arthritis: Comment on the article by Konig et al. *Ann. Rheum. Dis.* **2014**, *74*, e7. [CrossRef]
163. Kobayashi, T.; Ito, S.; Kobayashi, D.; Shimada, A.; Narita, I.; Murasawa, A.; Nakazono, K.; Yoshie, H. Serum Immunoglobulin G Levels to Porphyromonas gingivalis Peptidylarginine Deiminase Affect Clinical Response

to Biological Disease-Modifying Antirheumatic Drug in Rheumatoid Arthritis. *PLoS ONE* **2016**, *11*, e0154182. [CrossRef]
164. Shimada, A.; Kobayashi, T.; Ito, S.; Okada, M.; Murasawa, A.; Nakazono, K.; Yoshie, H. Expression of anti-Porphyromonas gingivalis peptidylarginine deiminase immunoglobulin G and peptidylarginine deiminase-4 in patients with rheumatoid arthritis and periodontitis. *J. Periodontal Res.* **2016**, *51*, 103–111. [CrossRef]
165. Vossenaar, E.R.; Nijenhuis, S.; Helsen, M.M.A.; Van Der Heijden, A.; Senshu, T.; Berg, W.B.V.D.; Van Venrooij, W.J.; Joosten, L.A.B. Citrullination of synovial proteins in murine models of rheumatoid arthritis. *Arthritis Rheum.* **2003**, *48*, 2489–2500. [CrossRef]
166. Cantaert, T.; Teitsma, C.; Tak, P.P.; Baeten, D. Presence and Role of Anti-Citrullinated Protein Antibodies in Experimental Arthritis Models. *Arthritis Rheum.* **2013**, *65*, 939–948. [CrossRef]
167. Konig, M.F.; Darrah, E.; Andrade, F. Insights into the significance of peptidylarginine deiminase 4 and antibodies against citrullinated antigens in the absence of "true ACPAs" in an experimental model of arthritis: Comment on the article by Shelef et al. *Arthritis Rheumatol.* **2014**, *66*, 2642–2644. [CrossRef]
168. Shelef, M.A.; Sokolove, J.; Robinson, W.H.; Huttenlocher, A. Insights into the significance of peptidylarginine deiminase 4 and antibodies against citrullinated antigens in the absence of "true ACPAs" in an experimental model of arthritis: Comment on the article by Shelef et al Reply. *Arthritis Rheumatol.* **2014**, *66*, 2644–2645. [CrossRef]
169. Vossenaar, E.R.; Van Boekel, M.A.M.; Van Venrooij, W.J.; López-Hoyoz, M.; Merino, J.; Merino, R.; Joosten, L.A.B. Absence of citrulline-specific autoantibodies in animal models of autoimmunity. *Arthritis Rheum.* **2004**, *50*, 2370–2372. [CrossRef]
170. Kingler, R. Untersuchungen über menschliche Aktinomycose. *Zent. Bakteriol* **1912**, *62*, 191–200.
171. Potts, T.V.; Zambon, J.J.; Genco, R.J. Reassignment of Actinobacillus-Actinomycetemcomitans to the Genus Hemophilus as Haemophilus-Actinomycetemcomitans Comb-Nov. *Int. J. Syst. Bacteriol.* **1985**, *35*, 337–341. [CrossRef]
172. Norskov-Lauritsen, N.; Kilian, M. Reclassification of *Actinobacillus actinomycetemcomitans*, Haemophilus aphrophilus, Haemophilus paraphrophilus and Haemophilus segnis as *Aggregatibacter actinomycetemcomitans* gen. nov., comb. nov., *Aggregatibacter aphrophilus* comb. nov. and Aggregatibacter segnis comb. nov., and emended description of Aggregatibacter aphrophilus to include V factor-dependent and V factor-independent isolates. *Int. J. Syst. Evol. Microbiol.* **2006**, *56*, 2135–2146.
173. Heinrich, S.; Pulverer, G. Zur Ätiologie und Mikrobiologie der Aktinomykose III. Die pathogene Bedeutung des Actinobacillus actinomycetem-comitans unter den "Begleitbakterien" des Actinomyces israeli. *Zent. Bakteriol* **1959**, *176*, 91–101.
174. Colebrook, L. The mycelial and other micro-organisms associated with human actinomycosis. *Br. J. Exp. Pathol.* **1920**, *1*, 197–212.
175. King, E.O.; Tatum, H.W. Actinobacillus Actinomycetemcomitans and Hemophilus Aphrophilus. *J. Infect. Dis.* **1962**, *111*, 85–94. [CrossRef]
176. Mitchell, R.G.; Gillespie, W.A. Bacterial endocarditis due to an actinobacillus. *J. Clin. Pathol.* **1964**, *17*, 511–512. [CrossRef]
177. Page, M.I.; King, E.O. Infection Due to Actinobacillus Actinomycetemcomitans and Haemophilus Aphrophilus. *N. Engl. J. Med.* **1966**, *275*, 181–188. [CrossRef]
178. Geraci, J.E.; Wilson, W.R. Symposium on infective endocarditis. III. Endocarditis due to gram-negative bacteria. Report of 56 cases. *Mayo Clin. Proc.* **1982**, *57*, 145–148.
179. Kaplan, A.H.; Weber, D.J.; Oddone, E.Z.; Perfect, J.R. Infection Due to Actinobacillus-Actinomycetemcomitans - 15 Cases and Review. *Rev. Infect. Dis.* **1989**, *11*, 46–63. [CrossRef]
180. van Winkelhoff, A.J.; Slots, J. Actinobacillus actinomycetemcomitans and Porphyromonas gingivalis in nonoral infections. *Periodontol. 2000.* **1999**, *20*, 122–135. [CrossRef]
181. Tanner, A.C.R.; Haffer, C.; Bratthall, G.T.; Visconti, R.A.; Socransky, S.S. A study of the bacteria associated with advancing periodontitis in man. *J. Clin. Periodontol.* **1979**, *6*, 278–307. [CrossRef]
182. Slots, J.; Reynolds, H.S.; Genco, R.J. Actinobacillus actinomycetemcomitans in Human Periodontal Disease: A Cross-Sectional Microbiological Investigation. *Infect. Immun.* **1980**, *29*, 1013–1020.

183. Zambon, J.J.; Christersson, L.A.; Slots, J. Actinobacillus actinomycetemcomitans in human periodontal disease. Prevalence in patient groups and distribution of biotypes and serotypes within families. *J. Periodontol.* **1983**, *54*, 707–711. [CrossRef]
184. Zambon, J.J.; Slots, J.; Genco, R.J. Serology of oral Actinobacillus actinomycetemcomitans and serotype distribution in human periodontal disease. *Infect. Immun.* **1983**, *41*, 19–27.
185. Slots, J.; Bragd, L.; Wikström, M.; Dahlén, G. The occurrence of Actinobacillus actinomycetemcomitans, Bacteroides gingivalis and Bacteroides intermedius in destructive periodontal disease in adults. *J. Clin. Periodontol.* **1986**, *13*, 570–577. [CrossRef]
186. Johansson, A. Aggregatibacter actinomycetemcomitans leukotoxin: A powerful tool with capacity to cause imbalance in the host inflammatory response. *Toxins (Basel)* **2011**, *3*, 242–259. [CrossRef]
187. Claesson, R.; Höglund-Åberg, C.; Haubek, D.; Johansson, A. Age-related prevalence and characteristics of Aggregatibacter actinomycetemcomitans in periodontitis patients living in Sweden. *J. Oral Microbiol.* **2017**, *9*, 1334504. [CrossRef]
188. Zambon, J.J. Actinobacillus actinomycetemcomitans in human periodontal disease. *J. Clin. Periodontol.* **1985**, *12*, 1–20. [CrossRef]
189. Chen, C.; Wang, T.; Chen, W. Occurrence of Aggregatibacter actinomycetemcomitans serotypes in subgingival plaque from United States subjects. *Mol. Oral Microbiol.* **2010**, *25*, 207–214. [CrossRef]
190. Pahumunto, N.; Ruangsri, P.; Wongsuwanlert, M.; Piwat, S.; Dahlén, G.; Teanpaisan, R. Aggregatibacter actinomycetemcomitans serotypes and DGGE subtypes in Thai adults with chronic periodontitis. *Arch. Oral Biol.* **2015**, *60*, 1789–1796. [CrossRef]
191. Kim, T.S.; Frank, P.; Eickholz, P.; Eick, S.; Kim, C.K. Serotypes of Aggregatibacter actinomycetemcomitans in patients with different ethnic backgrounds. *J. Periodontol.* **2009**, *80*, 2020–2027. [CrossRef]
192. Mínguez, M.; Pousa, X.; Herrera, D.; Blasi, A.; Sánchez, M.C.; León, R.; Sanz, M. Characterization and serotype distribution of Aggregatibacter actinomycetemcomitans isolated from a population of periodontitis patients in Spain. *Arch. Oral Biol.* **2014**, *59*, 1359–1367. [CrossRef]
193. Yang, H.W.; Huang, Y.F.; Chan, Y.; Chou, M.Y. Relationship of Actinobacillus actinomycetemcomitans serotypes to periodontal condition: Prevalence and proportions in subgingival plaque. *Eur. J. Oral Sci.* **2005**, *113*, 28–33. [CrossRef]
194. Arenas Rodrigues, V.A.; de Avila, E.D.; Nakano, V.; Avila-Campos, M.J. Qualitative, quantitative and genotypic evaluation of Aggregatibacter actinomycetemcomitans and Fusobacterium nucleatum isolated from individuals with different periodontal clinical conditions. *Anaerobe* **2018**, *52*, 50–58. [CrossRef]
195. Åberg, C.H.; Haubek, D.; Kwamin, F.; Johansson, A.; Claesson, R. Leukotoxic Activity of Aggregatibacter actinomycetemcomitans and Periodontal Attachment Loss. *PLoS ONE* **2014**, *9*, e104095.
196. Aberg, C.H.; Kelk, P.; Johansson, A. Aggregatibacter actinomycetemcomitans: Virulence of its leukotoxin and association with aggressive periodontitis. *Virulence* **2015**, *6*, 188–195. [CrossRef]
197. Linhartová, I.; Bumba, L.; Mašín, J.; Basler, M.; Osička, R.; Kamanová, J.; Procházková, K.; Adkins, I.; Hejnová-Holubová, J.; Sadílková, L.; et al. RTX proteins: A highly diverse family secreted by a common mechanism. *FEMS Microbiol. Rev.* **2010**, *34*, 1076–1112. [CrossRef]
198. Reinholdt, J.; Poulsen, K.; Brinkmann, C.R.; Hoffmann, S.V.; Stapulionis, R.; Enghild, J.J.; Jensen, U.B.; Boesen, T.; Vorup-Jensen, T. Monodisperse and LPS-free Aggregatibacter actinomycetemcomitans leukotoxin: Interactions with human beta2 integrins and erythrocytes. *Biochim. Biophys. Acta* **2013**, *1834*, 546–558. [CrossRef]
199. Brogan, J.M.; Lally, E.T.; Poulsen, K.; Kilian, M.; DeMuth, D.R. Regulation of Actinobacillus actinomycetemcomitans leukotoxin expression: Analysis of the promoter regions of leukotoxic and minimally leukotoxic strains. *Infect. Immun.* **1994**, *62*, 501–508.
200. Zambon, J.J.; Haraszthy, V.I.; Hariharan, G.; Lally, E.T.; DeMuth, D.R. The Microbiology of early-onset periodontitis: Association of highly toxic Actinobacillus actinomycetemcomitans strains with localized juvenile periodontitis. *J. Periodontol.* **1996**, *67*, 282–290. [CrossRef]
201. Sampathkumar, V.; Velusamy, S.K.; Godboley, D.; Fine, D.H. Increased leukotoxin production: Characterization of 100 base pairs within the 530 base pair leukotoxin promoter region of Aggregatibacter actinomycetemcomitans. *Sci. Rep.* **2017**, *7*, 1887. [CrossRef]

202. Burgess, D.; Huang, H.; Harrison, P.; Aukhil, I.; Shaddox, L. Aggregatibacter actinomycetemcomitans in African Americans with Localized Aggressive Periodontitis. *JDR Clin. Transl. Res.* **2017**, *2*, 249–257. [CrossRef]

203. Oscarsson, J.; Claesson, R.; Lindholm, M.; Höglund Åberg, C.; Johansson, A. Tools of Aggregatibacter actinomycetemcomitans to Evade the Host Response. *J. Clin. Med.* **2019**, *8*, 1079. [CrossRef]

204. Harvey, G.P.; Fitzsimmons, T.R.; Dhamarpatni, A.A.; Marchant, C.; Haynes, D.R.; Bartold, P.M. Expression of peptidylarginine deiminase-2 and -4, citrullinated proteins and anti-citrullinated protein antibodies in human gingiva. *J. Periodontal Res.* **2013**, *48*, 252–261. [CrossRef]

205. Nesse, W.; Westra, J.; van der Wal, J.E.; Abbas, F.; Nicholas, A.P.; Vissink, A.; Brouwer, E. The periodontium of periodontitis patients contains citrullinated proteins which may play a role in ACPA (anti-citrullinated protein antibody) formation. *J. Clin. Periodontol.* **2012**, *39*, 599–607. [CrossRef]

206. Malinin, T.I.; Pekin, T.J.; Zvaifler, N.J. Cytology of Synovial Fluid in Rheumatoid Arthritis. *Am. J. Clin. Pathol.* **1967**, *47*, 203–208. [CrossRef]

207. Darrah, E.; Rosen, A.; Giles, J.T.; Andrade, F. Peptidylarginine deiminase 2, 3 and 4 have distinct specificities against cellular substrates: Novel insights into autoantigen selection in rheumatoid arthritis. *Ann. Rheum. Dis.* **2012**, *71*, 92–98. [CrossRef]

208. Delima, A.J.; Van Dyke, T.E. Origin and function of the cellular components in gingival crevice fluid. *Periodontol 2000* **2003**, *31*, 55–76. [CrossRef]

209. Konig, M.F.; Andrade, F. A critical reappraisal of neutrophil extracellular traps (NETs) and NETosis mimics based on differential requirements for protein citrullination. *Front. Immunol.* **2016**, *7*, 461. [CrossRef]

210. Volkov, M.; Dekkers, J.; Loos, B.G.; Bizzarro, S.; Huizinga, T.W.J.; Praetorius, H.A.; Toes, R.E.M.; Van Der Woude, D. Comment on Aggregatibacter actinomycetemcomitans—Induced hypercitrullination links periodontal infection to autoimmunity in rheumatoid arthritis. *Sci. Transl. Med.* **2018**, *10*, eaan8349. [CrossRef]

211. Mukherjee, A.; Jantsch, V.; Khan, R.; Hartung, W.; Fischer, R.; Jantsch, J.; Ehrenstein, B.; Konig, M.F.; Andrade, F. Rheumatoid Arthritis-Associated Autoimmunity Due to Aggregatibacter actinomycetemcomitans and Its Resolution with Antibiotic Therapy. *Front. Immunol.* **2018**, *9*, 2352. [CrossRef]

212. Konig, M.F.; Giles, J.T.; Teles, R.P.; Moutsopoulos, N.M.; Andrade, F. Response to comment on "Aggregatibacter actinomycetemcomitans–induced hypercitrullination links periodontal infection to autoimmunity in rheumatoid arthritis". *Sci. Transl. Med.* **2018**, *10*, eaao3031. [CrossRef]

213. Queiroz-Junior, C.M.; Madeira, M.F.M.; Coelho, F.M.; Oliveira, C.R.; Cândido, L.C.M.; Garlet, G.P.; Teixeira, M.M.; Souza, D.D.G.; Da Silva, T.A.; Queiroz-Junior, C.M. Experimental arthritis exacerbates Aggregatibacter actinomycetemcomitans-induced periodontitis in mice. *J. Clin. Periodontol.* **2012**, *39*, 608–616. [CrossRef]

214. Taichman, N.S.; Shenker, B.J.; Tsai, C.C.; Glickman, L.T.; Baehni, P.C.; Stevens, R.; Hammond, B.F. Cytopathic effects of Actinobacillus actinomycetemcomitans on monkey blood leukocytes. *J. Periodontal Res.* **1984**, *19*, 133–145. [CrossRef]

215. Rantapää-Dahlqvist, S.; De Jong, B.A.W.; Berglin, E.; Hallmans, G.; Wadell, G.; Stenlund, H.; Sundin, U.; Van Venrooij, W.J. Antibodies against cyclic citrullinated peptide and IgA rheumatoid factor predict the development of rheumatoid arthritis. *Arthritis Rheum.* **2003**, *48*, 2741–2749. [CrossRef]

216. Nielen, M.M.J.; Van Schaardenburg, D.; Reesink, H.W.; Van De Stadt, R.J.; Van Der Horst-Bruinsma, I.E.; De Koning, M.H.M.T.; Habibuw, M.R.; Vandenbroucke, J.P.; Dijkmans, B.A.C.; Van Der Horst-Bruinsma, I.E. Specific autoantibodies precede the symptoms of rheumatoid arthritis: A study of serial measurements in blood donors. *Arthritis Rheum.* **2004**, *50*, 380–386. [CrossRef]

217. Makrygiannakis, D.; Klint, E.A.; Lundberg, I.E.; Lofberg, R.; Ulfgren, A.K.; Klareskog, L.; Catrina, A.I. Citrullination is an inflammation-dependent process. *Ann. Rheum. Dis.* **2006**, *65*, 1219–1222. [CrossRef]

218. Ramseier, C.A.; Anerud, A.; Dulac, M.; Lulic, M.; Cullinan, M.P.; Seymour, G.J.; Faddy, M.J.; Bürgin, W.; Schätzle, M.; Lang, N.P. Natural history of periodontitis: Disease progression and tooth loss over 40 years. *J. Clin. Periodontol.* **2017**, *44*, 1182–1191. [CrossRef]

219. Dal, P.M.; van der Goot, F.G. Pore-forming toxins: Ancient, but never really out of fashion. *Nat. Rev. Microbiol.* **2016**, *14*, 77–92.

220. Samuels, J.; Ng, Y.-S.; Coupillaud, C.; Paget, D.; Meffre, E. Impaired early B cell tolerance in patients with rheumatoid arthritis. *J. Exp. Med.* **2005**, *201*, 1659–1667. [CrossRef]

221. Samuels, J.; Ng, Y.S.; Coupillaud, C.; Paget, D.; Meffre, E. Human B cell tolerance and its failure in rheumatoid arthritis. *Ann. N. Y. Acad. Sci.* **2005**, *1062*, 116–126. [CrossRef]
222. Meffre, E.; Wardemann, H. B-cell tolerance checkpoints in health and autoimmunity. *Curr. Opin. Immunol.* **2008**, *20*, 632–638. [CrossRef]
223. Menard, L.; Samuels, J.; Ng, Y.S.; Meffre, E. Inflammation-independent defective early B cell tolerance checkpoints in rheumatoid arthritis. *Arthritis Rheum.* **2011**, *63*, 1237–1245. [CrossRef]
224. Borsotti, C.; Danzl, N.M.; Nauman, G.; Hölzl, M.A.; French, C.; Chavez, E.; Khosravi-Maharlooei, M.; Glauzy, S.; Delmotte, F.R.; Meffre, E.; et al. HSC extrinsic sex-related and intrinsic autoimmune disease–related human B-cell variation is recapitulated in humanized mice. *Blood Adv.* **2017**, *1*, 2007–2018. [CrossRef]
225. Marotte, H. Determining the Right Time for the Right Treatment—Application to Preclinical Rheumatoid Arthritis. *JAMA Netw. Open* **2019**, *2*, e195358. [CrossRef]
226. Kaur, S.; Bright, R.; Proudman, S.M.; Bartold, P.M. Does periodontal treatment influence clinical and biochemical measures for rheumatoid arthritis? A systematic review and meta-analysis. *Semin. Arthritis Rheum.* **2014**, *44*, 113–122. [CrossRef]
227. Monsarrat, P.; De Grado, G.F.; Constantin, A.; Willmann, C.; Nabet, C.; Sixou, M.; Cantagrel, A.; Barnetche, T.; Mehsen-Cetre, N.; Schaeverbeke, T.; et al. The effect of periodontal treatment on patients with rheumatoid arthritis: The ESPERA randomised controlled trial. *Jt. Bone Spine* **2019**, in press. [CrossRef]
228. Bright, R.; Thiele, G.M.; Manavis, J.; Mikuls, T.R.; Payne, J.B.; Bartold, P.M. Gingival tissue, an extrasynovial source of malondialdehyde-acetaldehyde adducts, citrullinated and carbamylated proteins. *J. Periodontal Res.* **2018**, *53*, 139–143. [CrossRef]
229. Darrah, E.; Andrade, F. Editorial: citrullination, and carbamylation, and malondialdehyde-acetaldehyde! Oh my! Entering the forest of autoantigen modifications in rheumatoid arthritis. *Arthritis Rheumatol.* **2015**, *67*, 604–608. [CrossRef]
230. Henle, J. *Von den Miasmen und Kontagien: Und Von den Miasmatisch-Kontagiösen Krankheiten (1840)*; Verlag von J. A. Barth: Leipzig, Germany, 1910.
231. Koch, R. Über Bakteriologische Forschung. In *Verhandlungen des X*; Internationalen Medicinischen Congresses: Berlin, Germany, 1890; Volume 1.
232. Rivers, T.M. Viruses and Koch's postulates. *J. Bacteriol.* **1937**, *33*, 1–12.
233. Correa, M.G.; Sacchetti, S.B.; Ribeiro, F.V.; Pimentel, S.P.; Casarin, R.C.V.; Cirano, F.R.; Casati, M.Z. Periodontitis increases rheumatic factor serum levels and citrullinated proteins in gingival tissues and alter cytokine balance in arthritic rats. *PLoS ONE* **2017**, *12*, e0174442. [CrossRef]

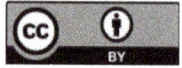

© 2019 by the authors. Licensee MDPI, Basel, Switzerland. This article is an open access article distributed under the terms and conditions of the Creative Commons Attribution (CC BY) license (http://creativecommons.org/licenses/by/4.0/).

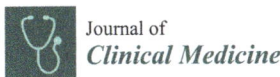

Review

Periodontitis: A Multifaceted Disease of Tooth-Supporting Tissues

Eija Könönen [1,2,*], Mervi Gursoy [1] and Ulvi Kahraman Gursoy [1]

1. Department of Periodontology, Institute of Dentistry, University of Turku, 20520 Turku, Finland
2. Oral Health Care, Welfare Division, City of Turku, 20101 Turku, Finland
* Correspondence: eija.kononen@utu.fi; Tel.: +358-50-4067-374

Received: 28 June 2019; Accepted: 29 July 2019; Published: 31 July 2019

Abstract: Periodontitis is an infection-driven inflammatory disease in which the composition of biofilms plays a significant role. Dental plaque accumulation at the gingival margin initiates an inflammatory response that, in turn, causes microbial alterations and may lead to drastic consequences in the periodontium of susceptible individuals. Chronic inflammation affects the gingiva and can proceed to periodontitis, which characteristically results in irreversible loss of attachment and alveolar bone. Periodontitis appears typically in adult-aged populations, but young individuals can also experience it and its harmful outcome. Advanced disease is the major cause of tooth loss in adults. In addition, periodontitis is associated with many chronic diseases and conditions affecting general health.

Keywords: periodontal disease; alveolar bone loss; gingiva; bacteria; biofilm; immunity; inflammation; smoking

1. Introduction

Periodontitis is an infection-driven inflammatory disease in tooth-supporting tissues (i.e., the periodontium). Moreover, genetics and environmental and behavioral factors are involved in the development of the disease, the exposure of susceptible individuals to its initiation, and the speed of progression. The structure of the periodontium is diverse; it is composed of the gingiva, the underlying connective tissue, cement on the root surface, alveolar bone, and the periodontal ligament between the cementum and alveolar bone (Figure 1A,B). The junctional epithelium of the gingiva is a unique structure, located at the bottom of the gingival sulcus, which controls the constant presence of bacteria at this site. The most characteristic feature of periodontitis is the activation of osteoclastogenesis and the destruction of alveolar bone as its consequence, which is irreversible and leads to loss of tooth support.

Periodontal disease, especially its mild and moderate forms, is highly prevalent in adult-aged populations all over the world, with prevalence rates around 50% [1], while its severe form increases especially between the third and fourth decades of life, with the global prevalence being around 10% [2]. Certain demographic characteristics, such as age, gender, ethnicity, and socioeconomic status, influence the prevalence of periodontitis. Other strongly contributing factors include smoking, diabetes mellitus, metabolic syndrome, and obesity [3,4]. It is noteworthy that smoking and diabetes can expose individuals to the advanced form of periodontal disease already in adolescence and early adulthood [5–7]. There is also a strong relation of smoking to tooth loss in young individuals [8]. Severe periodontitis, the major cause of tooth loss in adults (https://www.nidcr.nih.gov/research/data-statistics/periodontal-disease), is typically complicated by the drifting and hypermobility of teeth, eventually resulting in the collapsed bite function of an affected individual [9,10]. Moreover, periodontal disease as well as tooth loss are considered to have an association with a variety of chronic diseases and conditions affecting general health.

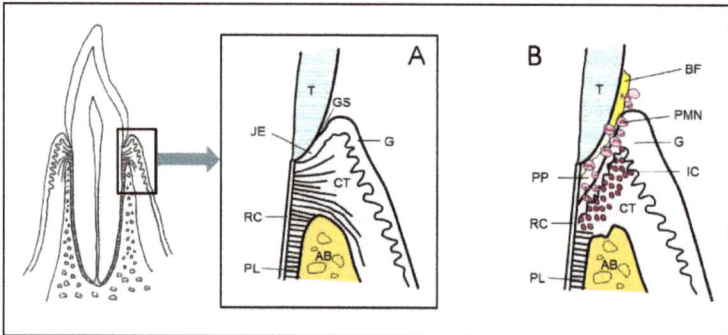

Figure 1. The anatomical structure of the periodontium in health (**A**) and in periodontitis (**B**). Abbreviations: Alveolar bone (AB), bacterial biofilm (BF), connective tissue (CT), gingiva (G), gingival sulcus (GS), inflammatory cells (IC), junctional epithelium (JE), polymorphonuclear neutrophils (PMN), periodontal ligament (PL), periodontal pocket (PP), root cementum (RC), and tooth (T).

Even in periodontal health, immune cells are constantly present in the gingiva, thus supporting the balance between oral biofilms and the host [11]. This constant communication keeps the immune response active, being a reciprocal, synergistic, and dynamic interaction. In the periodontium, the immune response carries characteristics of that of any other part of the body; the first action against microbes is due to non-specific innate response, while extended pathogenic challenge activates specific adaptive responses.

Excessive dental plaque accumulation at the gingival margin leads to inflammation and increasing proportions of proteolytic and often obligately anaerobic species [12]. The presence of periodontal species with pathogenic potential in the gingival sulcus initiates an inflammatory response in gingival tissue. When allowed to become chronic, this can have drastic consequences in the periodontium of susceptible individuals. Interactions between the components and metabolic activities of the oral microbiota and the host either support the balance (homeostasis) or result in disturbance (dysbiosis) within the microbiota [12]. Periodontal health-associated commensals are important in protecting the balance, for example, by inhibiting the growth of periodontitis-associated pathogens. However, qualitative and quantitative alterations within subgingival biofilms can result in disrupted homeostasis, which consequently can lead to the onset of disease with various degrees of periodontal tissue destruction.

2. Pathogenic Biofilms

Multispecies biofilm formation and maturation occur on tooth surfaces via intergeneric interactions, where coaggregations occur between different bacterial taxa, and highly diverse bacterial communities are formed at supragingival (above the gumline) and subgingival (below the gumline) sites [13,14]. *Fusobacterium nucleatum*, which belongs to the core anaerobic microbiota of the oral cavity from early years of life onwards [15,16], is seen as an important bridging organism of maturing dental biofilms, allowing late-colonizing species with virulent properties to be colonized [13]. This gradual maturation and shifts in the microbial composition influence the pathogenicity of subgingival biofilms where metabolically highly specialized microorganisms function in physical proximity as interactive microbial communities [12]. Focusing on only its adherence capabilities may lead to the underestimation of other important virulence characteristics of *F. nucleatum*, a relevant bacterium in the initiation and progression of periodontal disease. In a biofilm, this obligate anaerobe can survive and increase its numbers in aerobic environments [17]. Indeed, recent evidence indicates that *F. nucleatum* induces an environmental change through hypoxia [18], which can support the colonization of anaerobic pathogens in dental biofilms. The effects of *F. nucleatum*-induced hypoxia are not limited to the shifts in the biofilm composition—this hypoxia also directs endothelial cells to an inflammatory state and activates angiogenesis [18].

In subgingival biofilms, anaerobic gram-negative species with their biologically active lipopolysaccharide (LPS)-containing cell wall structure may be essential in awakening the inflammatory reaction in the gingiva and culprits of periodontal destruction to occur in periodontitis-susceptible individuals [11]. Subgingival plaque samples collected from periodontitis patients and periodontitis-free individuals differ from each other. *Porphyromonas gingivalis*, *Tannerella forsythia*, and *Treponema denticola*, the so-called red complex, have shown the strongest association with periodontal disease [19]. In another study by using 454 pyrosequencing of 16S rRNA genes, *P. gingivalis* and *T. denticola* but also *Filifactor alocis*, a gram-positive anaerobe, formed the top three species [20]. Of these, *P. gingivalis* is suggested to be the principal pathogen in the process, causing a disturbed interplay between the subgingival biofilm and the host response [21]. Even as a minor constituent of the subgingival microbiota, it is able to severely affect the ecosystem by influencing the numbers and community organization of commensal bacteria at the site and dysregulate innate immunity pathways. *P. gingivalis*, a highly proteolytic gram-negative anaerobe, is a common recovery from deepened periodontal pockets of adult periodontitis patients. While *P. gingivalis* is rather rare in children and adolescents, its salivary carriage rates increase significantly with aging, and it is detected in the majority of the Finnish population after the age of 55 years [22]. Different from *P. gingivalis*, the carriage of *Aggregatibacter actinomycetemcomitans* was less frequent, without any connection to age. This gram-negative capnophilic coccobacillus and an established periodontal pathogen has been linked to aggressive forms of periodontal disease [23]. Besides these traditional pathogens, open-ended molecular methods have significantly enlarged the list of pathogenic species within periodontitis-associated subgingival biofilms [24].

Many periodontitis-associated species, among those *A. actinomycetemcomitans*, *P. gingivalis*, and *F. nucleatum*, or even polymicrobial aggregates, are capable of invading periodontal tissues [25–27], thus evading many defense mechanisms of the host. This, in turn, has an impact on the persistence of inflammation and progression of periodontal tissue destruction.

For periodontal disease to occur, it is not the presence of a single periodontal pathogen, but the interplay between the composition of the subgingival biofilm and the host response where host factors and specific niches play an important role. In dysbiotic biofilms, there is abundance of immunostimulatory pathobionts and their virulence factors, but also a reduced inhibitory effect of commensal bacteria, thus resulting in an increased inflammatory response [28,29]. In gingival epithelia, cellular responses are especially elicited against polymicrobial biofilms due to their interbacterial metabolic and virulence synergisms [30], leading the way to initial pocket formation and attachment loss. Deepening periodontal pockets with an anaerobic environment, inflammatory conditions, and a large amount of substrates originating from tissue destruction all favor the growth of inflammophilic periodontal pathogens and pathobionts [21]. Notably, daily smoking contributes to further disturbances in the subgingival microbiota, facilitating an abundance of periodontal pathogens and the reduction of beneficial commensals, thus exposing smokers to periodontal disease [31].

There have been intensive research activities targeting periodontitis-associated bacteria and/or the antibodies working against them, with the aim of revealing their involvement in various systemic diseases and conditions. Major periodontal pathogens raise local and systemic antibody responses; it has been shown in multivariate analyses that the main determinant of the systemic antibody response to *P. gingivalis* and *A. actinomycetemcomitans* is the carriage of the pathogen, whereas the presence or degree of periodontal disease has only a modest modifying effect [32]. High serum IgG antibodies to major periodontal pathogens act as risk factors for future cardiovascular events [33–35]. Also, the circulation of LPS of virulent gram-negative pathogens (endotoxemia) accompanied by exaggerated proinflammatory responses is connected to risk for these events [33]. Subgingival bacteria, including *P. gingivalis* and *A. actinomycetemcomitans*, have also been associated with the prevalence of prediabetes in young diabetes-free adults [36]. Interestingly, associations between bacterial measures and prediabetes are consistently stronger than those between periodontitis and prediabetes. Furthermore, there is accumulating evidence on the role of *P. gingivalis* in rheumatoid arthritis [37,38]. A prospective study on the association between pancreatic cancer and the oral microbiome revealed that the carriage of *P. gingivalis* and *A. actinomycetemcomitans* is a subsequent risk for this highly lethal cancer type [39]. Besides the impact of *F. nucleatum* as the key organism in dental biofilms and its involvement in oral and extra-oral polymicrobial infections [40], recent research has shown its significant carcinogenic potential. Its ability to tolerate oxygen, create hypoxia, and induce an inflammatory environment may explain the role of *F. nucleatum* in the development and progression of colorectal adenocarcinoma [41].

3. Immunologic Players of the Periodontium

Due to the constant interaction with bacteria, immune cells (neutrophils, macrophages, and lymphocytes) are present in the periodontium to take part in maintaining a healthy equilibrium. Neutrophils continuously transmigrate through the junctional epithelium to gingival sulcus and release antimicrobial peptides (α-defensins) against invading bacteria, while they also stimulate adhesion and the spread of keratinocytes on the tooth surface [42]. Resident cells of the periodontium (keratinocytes, fibroblasts, dendritic cells, and osteoblasts) are not passive barriers against bacterial invasion, but they initiate innate immune response and regulate adaptive immune response [43,44]. An essential component is the complement pathway, which activates, amplifies, and synchronizes innate immune response by opsonizing and killing bacteria as well as activating mast cells, neutrophils, and macrophages of the periodontium [45].

Keratinocytes, which form the majority of the gingival epithelium, are capable of producing and secreting various immune response mediators, among them human β-defensins (hBDs), cathelicidins, proinflammatory cytokines, chemokines, and angiogenetic proteins [46,47]. In the healthy gingiva, innate response is mainly regulated by keratinocytes and neutrophils; keratinocytes secrete hBDs to protect the oral and sulcular epithelium (Figure 2A), whereas neutrophils secrete α-defensins to protect the junctional epithelium (Figure 2B). Gingival keratinocytes recognize pathogen-associated molecular patterns (PAMPs) by their pattern recognition receptors, such as toll-like receptors (TLRs). mRNA expressions of TLR 1–9 are detected in connective tissue and epithelial layers of the gingiva [48]. In addition, bacterial signaling molecules (cyclic dinucleotides and quorum signaling molecules) activate cytokine response in gingival keratinocytes [49,50]. There is also a reciprocal interaction between innate-immune proteins and keratinocytes. For example, proinflammatory interleukins (IL-1α, IL-1β, IL-6) activate the protein expression and secretion of hBDs from keratinocytes [46,51], while keratinocytes can suppress the inflammatory response by secreting monocyte chemotactic protein-induced protein-1 [52].

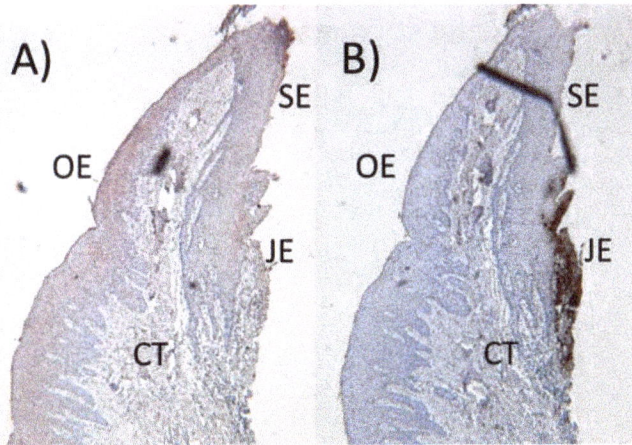

Figure 2. In a healthy gingiva, epithelial defensins (human β-defensins (hBD-2) in red color) are located in the oral (OE) and sulcular (SE) epithelia (**A**), while neutrophilic antimicrobial peptides (α-defensins in brown color) are located in the junctional epithelium (JE) and partly in connective tissue (CT) (**B**). (An original figure by U.K.G.)

Gingival connective tissue, periodontal ligament, and the organic component of the bone are formed of collagen. Fibroblasts are responsible for the synthesis of new collagen bundles and they remove the old collagen by secreting matrix metalloproteinases (MMPs). Overexpression of MMPs by gingival fibroblasts may either induce the release of cytokines and chemokines from the extracellular matrix or cleave cytokines and interrupt immune response signaling cascades [53]. The interplay between neutrophils and gingival fibroblasts is a good example of the bidirectional interactions between resident and immune cells.

Dendritic cells differ from keratinocytes and fibroblasts by acting as phagocytes and antigen-presenting cells. In a healthy environment, dendritic cells are in their immature forms and have high phagocytic capacity against invading microorganisms, but during infection they initiate a maturation process that involves their migration to lymph nodes to activate $CD4^+$ T cells [54] and promote the polarization of T-helper (Th)1, Th2, Th17, and B cells [55]. Uncontrolled upregulation of Th1 and Th17 cell pathways enhances alveolar bone loss via the induction of osteoclastogenesis [56]. There is also evidence that dendritic cells can differentiate to osteoclasts [57]; however, it is unknown how much of the bone resorption seen in periodontitis is actually induced by dendritic cell-derived osteoclasts.

Neutrophils form the primary defense system in periodontal tissues. Notably, their migration through the junctional epithelium into the gingival sulcus is a continuous process, which may differ from other organs, where transmigration is a hallmark of infection [58]. In the healthy oral cavity, neutrophil populations tend to be parainflammatory, while proinflammatory neutrophil phenotypes are present in periodontal disease [59]. Severe forms of periodontitis can be connected to diseases with neutrophil function defects, such as leukocyte adhesion deficiency 1 (LAD-1). Lack of neutrophil surveillance against bacterial infection is considered the cause of excessive periodontal degradation in neutrophil function deficiencies. However, recent evidence indicates that the absence of neutrophils in LAD-1 leads to the overproduction of IL-17, which eventually enhances the proliferation and differentiation of B cells [60]. Chronic granulomatous disease (CGD) is another genetic disease, which is characterized by defective neutrophilic respiratory burst and bacterial elimination. Although CGD patients are prone to developing bacterial and fungal infections, their periodontitis prevalence does not differ from that of the general population. In the highlights of these two examples, the presence of neutrophils in the periodontal immune response cascade seems to be more important than their ability to kill bacteria, as other phagocytes can take care of bacterial killing [60]. Interestingly, peripheral blood neutrophils of periodontitis patients release higher levels of proinflammatory cytokines and reactive oxygen species compared to periodontally healthy individuals, and this hyperinflammatory response persists even after successful periodontal treatment [61,62].

Neutrophils have a relatively short lifespan and they are programmed to die via apoptosis. Apoptotic neutrophils are phagocytosed from tissues by macrophages and are eliminated through lymphatics (efferocytosis). Since neutrophils produce and secrete a significant number of inflammatory molecules, their removal is a hallmark of healing. In inflamed periodontal tissues, partly due to pathogenic biofilms, there is an extended recruitment of neutrophils and delayed apoptotic cell death [63]. Instead of enhanced elimination of pathogens, however, neutrophils demonstrate impaired antibacterial function with this uncontrolled and extended immune response activation [64].

Tissue macrophages derive either from circulating monocytes or from embryo-derived precursors [65]. Phenotyping them as inflammatory and resolving macrophages will define their roles in disease and health. Inflammatory macrophages produce and secrete a large group of cytokines (IL-1β, IL-23, IL-6, tumor necrosis factor (TNF)-α) and enzymes (MMPs) that take part in osteoclastogenesis and collagen degradation in periodontitis [66]. A conversion from a destructive inflammatory phenotype to a resolving and bone-forming phenotype requires both signaling molecules and the presence of apoptotic neutrophils [67]. *P. gingivalis* can reverse the conversion of inflammatory macrophages to resolving macrophages by inducing inflammatory cytokines [68]. Impaired elimination of neutrophils by macrophages and defects in the activation of resolving macrophages may in turn lead to the initiation and progression of periodontitis.

Innate immune cells present intra- and extracellular pathogens to lymphocytes. In the gingiva, the most common subset of lymphocytes is $CD4^+$ T cells, followed by $CD8^+$ T cells, which are further subgrouped as Th1, Th2, Th17, Th9, regulatory (Treg), and unconventional $\gamma\delta$ T cells [69]. Recent evidence indicates the role of Th17 cells as one main regulator of T cell response and bone resorption in the periodontium [70]. In addition, Treg cells can limit the progression of periodontal disease without suppressing the immune response. When chronic gingivitis progresses to periodontitis, there is a shift from T cell dominance to B and plasma cells. Different types of B cells include naive B cells, memory B cells, and antibody-secreting B cells. Antibodies produced against periodontitis-associated pathogens can be found in saliva and in serum as well [32].

Finally, periodontitis is a complex disease with a nonlinear character, and its effects on immune response are rather disproportional [71]. Although knowledge about immune cell functions has considerably increased, it is still difficult to fully understand cellular interactions in periodontal disease pathogenesis due to its multicausal etiology.

4. Inflammatory Process and Periodontal Tissue Destruction

The junctional epithelium forms a unique seal between the root surface and gingiva, and its main function is to provide protection to the underlying tissues against the constant exposure of oral microbes and their by-products [72]. Various molecular factors involved in adhesion, cell–cell interactions, chemotaxis, proinflammatory cytokines, epithelial growth, MMP activation, and antimicrobial peptide production contribute to the function of the junctional epithelium. If this elegant and well-adapted defense system is overwhelmed by bacterial virulence factors (e.g., *P. gingivalis* gingipains) and prolonged inflammation (clinically seen as gingival bleeding and changes in soft tissue contour and color), the junctional epithelium migrates apically on the root surface and activates collagen destruction, which eventually leads to periodontal pocket formation [72]. It is noteworthy that although gingival inflammation is the precursor of periodontitis and a clinically relevant risk factor for disease progression, not all gingivitis lesions lead to periodontitis [73]. During periodontal pocket formation, new tissue formation by resident cells (keratinocytes, fibroblasts, osteoblasts) is suppressed, whereas tissue degradation by neutrophils, macrophages, and osteoclasts is stimulated; thus, the balance between tissue removal and regeneration is disrupted [74].

Proinflammatory cytokines (IL-1β, IL-6, IL-23, TNF-α), chemokines (IL-8), and antimicrobial peptides produced by keratinocytes, fibroblasts, and dendritic cells are chemoattractant gradients for neutrophils, which migrate into inflamed tissues and stimulate the chemotaxis of nonresident cells (macrophages, lymphocytes, plasma cells, and mast cells) to the site of infection [43,44]. Phagocytic cells mainly aim to eliminate invading pathogens by producing and secreting antimicrobial agents, reactive oxygen species, and enzymes. However, abundant tissue concentrations of collagenolytic MMPs and elastase activate the degradation of type I collagen in the connective tissue and periodontal ligament [75]. During disease, MMP-8 is the major collagenase in periodontal tissues. Irreversible periodontal destruction occurs when the inflammatory cell infiltrate, predominantly containing plasma cells, extends deeper into the connective tissue, leading to tissue damage in periodontal ligament and alveolar bone [76].

Alveolar bone resorption is the principal pathological characteristic of periodontitis. The activation of osteoclasts, multi-nucleated bone-resorbing cells, is regulated by a cascade of inflammatory proteins (cytokines) and enzymes (MMPs). IL-1β, IL-6, and TNF-α are the major proinflammatory cytokines in osteoclastogenesis activation, which is achieved by upregulating the receptor of nuclear factor-kappa ligand (RANKL) expression and inhibiting the differentiation of osteoblasts as well as decreasing osteocalcin production and new bone formation [77]. Due to the upregulated RANKL (stimulator of mature osteoclast formation) and downregulated osteoprotegerin (blocker of RANKL action), degradation of the bone is enabled to progress. MMP-1, -8, and -13 are especially involved in alveolar bone destruction by degrading type I collagen (the main type of collagen in the periodontium), while two gelatinases (MMP-2 and -9) accomplish the degradation of denatured collagen [78]. Furthermore, MMP-9 assists in osteoclast migration and MMP-13 triggers osteoclast activation, which all facilitate type I collagen degradation.

The disease development with fast or slow progress and with stable periods varies among periodontal sites and among individuals. Diagnosis of periodontitis is based on clinical and radiographic information on periodontal attachment and alveolar bone loss. In the current classification system, staging estimates the severity of the disease, while grading aims to estimate the rate of its progression, taking the known risk factors into account [10]. At the early phase of periodontal disease, the clinical signs and symptoms can be lacking or very mild. When periodontal tissue destruction proceeds, deepened pocket depths with alveolar bone loss result in tooth mobility, drifting, flaring, and finally loss of the affected tooth. In advanced cases, where several teeth are affected, these abnormalities lead to the collapse of the bite function.

5. Periodontal Therapy—Impact on Oral and General Health

The primary goal of periodontal therapy is to reduce the infectious and inflammatory challenge and to halt the progressing tissue destruction. Removal of pathogenic biofilms and suppression of inflammation can discontinue the periodontal tissue degradation; however, only limited regain of lost tissues occurs, depending on the form of tissue defects, systemic health status, and age [79]. In advanced cases, the active anti-infective treatment phase is often combined with surgery to eliminate residual pockets—with the aim of improving the ecology at periodontal sites—or sometimes with adjunctive systemic antimicrobials to reduce pathogen burden. In smokers, however, the treatment outcome is compromised, which makes smoking cessation an essential part of their periodontal therapy [80,81]. The beneficial influence of quitting may partly be due to decreased pathogen numbers and increased abundance of health-associated commensals in subgingival biofilms [82]. Although anti-infective treatment reduces total bacterial counts, proportions of periodontal pathogens, as well as the number of sites colonized with pathogens, many of the species return with time [83]. Therefore, daily oral hygiene of the patient and continuing professional supportive periodontal therapy are necessary to maintain the outcome and strengthen the long-term success of the treatment [84,85]. Moreover, patients with advanced disease and masticatory dysfunction and bite collapse due to severe tooth loss have an obvious need for complex rehabilitation of the bite function as well as esthetic treatment. After treatment, however, periodontitis patients with prosthodontic reconstructions have still an increased risk for tooth loss, and many patient-related factors such as age, socioeconomic status, non-compliance, and diabetes are associated with abutment tooth loss [86].

Since untreated periodontitis increases systemic low-grade inflammation, another treatment goal is to improve this condition [87]. Although intensive mechanical periodontal treatment of patients with severely damaged periodontal tissues can cause an acute systemic inflammatory response and impair endothelial function, this occurs only transiently and, after six months, a significantly improved endothelial function is reached [88]. Furthermore, periodontal treatment has been shown to reduce atherosclerotic biomarkers (e.g., IL-6, TNF-α) of individuals with cardiovascular disease and/or diabetes [89] as well as to improve the glycemic status (Hba1c levels) of diabetic patients [90,91].

6. Future Considerations

Periodontal disease is multifactorial and the imbalance between tissue loss and gain can occur due to various reasons, including aggressive infection, uncontrolled chronic inflammation, weakened healing, or all of the above simultaneously. Thus, successful disease management requires an understanding of different elements of the disease at the individual level and the design of personalized treatment modalities, including immunotherapies and modulators of inflammation [92,93]. With the aid of newly developed omics technologies, these novel strategies may become available for clinicians.

Author Contributions: Conceptualization: E.K., U.K.G.; Writing: E.K., M.G., U.K.G.; Visualization: M.G., U.K.G.

Conflicts of Interest: The authors declare no conflict of interest.

References

1. Eke, P.I.; Dye, B.A.; Wei, L.; Thornton-Evans, G.O.; Genco, R.J. Prevalence of periodontitis in adults in the United States: 2009 and 2010. *J. Dent. Res.* **2012**, *91*, 914–920. [CrossRef] [PubMed]
2. Kassebaum, N.J.; Bernabé, E.; Dahiya, M.; Bhandari, B.; Murray, C.J.; Marcenes, W. Global burden of severe periodontitis in 1990–2010: A systematic review and meta-regression. *J. Dent. Res.* **2014**, *93*, 1045–1053. [CrossRef] [PubMed]
3. Genco, R.J.; Borgnakke, W.S. Risk factors for periodontal disease. *Periodontol. 2000* **2013**, *62*, 59–94. [CrossRef] [PubMed]
4. Lalla, E.; Papapanou, P.N. Diabetes mellitus and periodontitis: A tale of two common interrelated diseases. *Nat. Rev. Endocrinol.* **2011**, *7*, 738–748. [CrossRef] [PubMed]
5. Lalla, E.; Cheng, B.; Lal, S.; Kaplan, S.; Softness, B.; Greenberg, E.; Goland, R.S.; Lamster, I.B. Diabetes mellitus promotes periodontal destruction in children. *J. Clin. Periodontol.* **2007**, *34*, 294–298. [CrossRef] [PubMed]
6. Heikkinen, A.M.; Pajukanta, R.; Pitkäniemi, J.; Broms, U.; Sorsa, T.; Koskenvuo, M.; Meurman, J.H. The effect of smoking on periodontal health of 15- to 16-year-old adolescents. *J. Periodontol.* **2008**, *79*, 2042–2047. [CrossRef] [PubMed]
7. Thomson, W.M.; Shearer, D.M.; Broadbent, J.M.; Foster Page, L.A.; Poulton, R. The natural history of periodontal attachment loss during the third and fourth decades of life. *J. Clin. Periodontol.* **2013**, *40*, 672–680. [CrossRef] [PubMed]
8. Ylöstalo, P.; Sakki, T.; Laitinen, J.; Järvelin, M.R.; Knuuttila, M. The relation of tobacco smoking to tooth loss among young adults. *Eur. J. Oral Sci.* **2004**, *112*, 121–126. [CrossRef] [PubMed]
9. Kosaka, T.; Ono, T.; Yoshimuta, Y.; Kida, M.; Kikui, M.; Nokubi, T.; Maeda, Y.; Kokubo, Y.; Watanabe, M.; Miyamoto, Y. The effect of periodontal status and occlusal support on masticatory performance: The Suita study. *J. Clin. Periodontol.* **2014**, *41*, 497–503. [CrossRef]
10. Tonetti, M.S.; Greenwell, H.; Kornman, K.S. Staging and grading of periodontitis: Framework and proposal of a new classification and case definition. *J. Clin. Periodontol.* **2018**, *45* (Suppl. 20), S149–S161. [CrossRef]
11. Darveau, R.P. Periodontitis: A polymicrobial disruption of host homeostasis. *Nat. Rev. Microbiol.* **2010**, *8*, 481–490. [CrossRef] [PubMed]
12. Sanz, M.; Beighton, D.; Curtis, M.A.; Cury, J.A.; Dige, I.; Dommisch, H.; Ellwood, R.; Giacaman, R.A.; Herrera, D.; Herzberg, M.C.; et al. Role of microbial biofilms in the maintenance of oral health and in the

development of dental caries and periodontal diseases. Consensus report of group 1 of the joint EFP/ORCA workshop on the boundaries between caries and periodontal disease. *J. Clin. Periodontol.* **2017**, *44* (Suppl. 18), 5–11. [CrossRef] [PubMed]
13. Kolenbrander, P.E.; Palmer, R.J., Jr.; Periasamy, S.; Jakubovics, N.S. Oral multispecies biofilm development and the key role of cell-cell distance. *Nat. Rev. Microbiol.* **2010**, *8*, 471–480. [CrossRef] [PubMed]
14. Paster, B.J.; Boches, S.K.; Galvin, J.L.; Ericson, R.E.; Lau, C.N.; Levanos, V.A.; Sahasrabudhe, A.; Dewhirst, F.E. Bacterial diversity in human subgingival plaque. *J. Bacteriol.* **2001**, *183*, 3770–3783. [CrossRef]
15. Könönen, E. Development of oral bacterial flora in young children. *Ann. Med.* **2000**, *32*, 107–112. [CrossRef]
16. Haraldsson, G.; Holbrook, W.P.; Könönen, E. Clonal persistence of oral *Fusobacterium nucleatum* in infancy. *J. Dent. Res.* **2004**, *83*, 500–504. [CrossRef]
17. Gursoy, U.K.; Pöllänen, M.; Könönen, E.; Uitto, V.J. Biofilm formation enhances the oxygen tolerance and invasiveness of *Fusobacterium nucleatum* in an oral mucosa culture model. *J. Periodontol.* **2010**, *81*, 1084–1091. [CrossRef]
18. Mendes, R.T.; Nguyen, D.; Stephens, D.; Pamuk, F.; Fernandes, D.; Hasturk, H.; Van Dyke, T.E.; Kantarci, A. Hypoxia-induced endothelial cell responses - possible roles during periodontal disease. *Clin. Exp. Dent. Res.* **2018**, *4*, 241–248. [CrossRef]
19. Socransky, S.S.; Haffajee, A.D.; Cugini, M.A.; Smith, C.; Kent, R.L., Jr. Microbial complexes in subgingival plaque. *J. Clin. Periodontol.* **1998**, *25*, 134–144. [CrossRef]
20. Griffen, A.L.; Beall, C.J.; Campbell, J.H.; Firestone, N.D.; Kumar, P.S.; Yang, Z.K.; Podar, M.; Leys, E.J. Distinct and complex bacterial profiles in human periodontitis and health revealed by 16S pyrosequencing. *ISME J.* **2012**, *6*, 1176–1185. [CrossRef]
21. Hajishengallis, G. The inflammophilic character of the periodontitis-associated microbiota. *Mol. Oral Microbiol.* **2014**, *29*, 248–257. [CrossRef] [PubMed]
22. Könönen, E.; Paju, S.; Pussinen, P.J.; Hyvönen, M.; Di Tella, P.; Suominen-Taipale, L.; Knuuttila, M. Population-based study of salivary carriage of periodontal pathogens in adults. *J. Clin. Microbiol.* **2007**, *45*, 2446–2451. [CrossRef]
23. Könönen, E.; Müller, H.P. Microbiology of aggressive periodontitis. *Periodontol. 2000* **2014**, *65*, 46–78. [CrossRef] [PubMed]
24. Curtis, M.A. Periodontal microbiology - the lid's off the box again. *J. Dent. Res.* **2014**, *93*, 840–842. [CrossRef] [PubMed]
25. Saglie, F.R.; Marfany, A.; Camargo, P. Intragingival occurrence of *Actinobacillus actinomycetemcomitans* and *Bacteroides gingivalis* in active destructive periodontal lesions. *J. Periodontol.* **1988**, *59*, 259–265. [CrossRef] [PubMed]
26. Gursoy, U.K.; Könönen, E.; Uitto, V.J. Intracellular replication of fusobacteria requires new actin filament formation of epithelial cells. *APMIS* **2008**, *116*, 1063–1070. [CrossRef] [PubMed]
27. Baek, K.; Ji, S.; Choi, Y. Complex intratissue microbiota forms biofilms in periodontal lesions. *J. Dent. Res.* **2018**, *97*, 192–200. [CrossRef] [PubMed]
28. Jiao, Y.; Hasegawa, M.; Inohara, N. The role of oral pathobionts in dysbiosis during periodontitis development. *J. Dent. Res.* **2014**, *93*, 539–546. [CrossRef] [PubMed]
29. Herrero, E.R.; Fernandes, S.; Verspecht, T.; Ugarte-Berzal, E.; Boon, N.; Proost, P.; Bernaerts, K.; Quirynen, M.; Teughels, W. Dysbiotic biofilms deregulate the periodontal inflammatory response. *J. Dent. Res.* **2018**, *97*, 547–555. [CrossRef]
30. Peyyala, R.; Kirakodu, S.S.; Novak, K.F.; Ebersole, J.L. Oral microbial biofilm stimulation of epithelial cell responses. *Cytokine* **2012**, *58*, 65–72. [CrossRef]
31. Mason, M.R.; Preshaw, P.M.; Nagaraja, H.N.; Dabdoub, S.M.; Rahman, A.; Kumar, P.S. The subgingival microbiome of clinically healthy current and never smokers. *ISME J.* **2015**, *9*, 268–272. [CrossRef] [PubMed]
32. Pussinen, P.J.; Könönen, E.; Paju, S.; Hyvärinen, K.; Gursoy, U.K.; Huumonen, S.; Knuuttila, M.; Suominen, A.L. Periodontal pathogen carriage, rather than periodontitis, determines the serum antibody levels. *J. Clin. Periodontol.* **2011**, *38*, 405–411. [CrossRef] [PubMed]
33. Pussinen, P.J.; Tuomisto, K.; Jousilahti, P.; Havulinna, A.S.; Sundvall, J.; Salomaa, V. Endotoxemia, immune response to periodontal pathogens, and systemic inflammation associate with incident cardiovascular disease events. *Arterioscler. Thromb. Vasc. Biol.* **2007**, *27*, 1433–1439. [CrossRef] [PubMed]

34. Damgaard, C.; Reinholdt, J.; Enevold, C.; Fiehn, N.E.; Nielsen, C.H.; Holmstrup, P. Immunoglobulin G antibodies against *Porphyromonas gingivalis* or *Aggregatibacter actinomycetemcomitans* in cardiovascular disease and periodontitis. *J. Oral Microbiol.* **2017**, *9*, 1374154. [CrossRef] [PubMed]
35. Palm, F.; Lahdentausta, L.; Sorsa, T.; Tervahartiala, T.; Gokel, P.; Buggle, F.; Safer, A.; Becher, H.; Grau, A.J.; Pussinen, P. Biomarkers of periodontitis and inflammation in ischemic stroke: A case-control study. *Innate Immun.* **2014**, *20*, 511–518. [CrossRef]
36. Demmer, R.T.; Jacobs, D.R., Jr.; Singh, R.; Zuk, A.; Rosenbaum, M.; Papapanou, P.N.; Desvarieux, M. Periodontal bacteria and prediabetes prevalence in ORIGINS: The oral infections, glucose intolerance, and insulin resistance study. *J. Dent. Res.* **2015**, *94*, 201–211. [CrossRef]
37. Scher, J.U.; Ubeda, C.; Equinda, M.; Khanin, R.; Buischi, Y.; Viale, A.; Lipuma, L.; Attur, M.; Pillinger, M.H.; Weissmann, G.; et al. Periodontal disease and the oral microbiota in new-onset rheumatoid arthritis. *Arthritis Rheum.* **2012**, *64*, 3083–3094. [CrossRef]
38. Eriksson, K.; Fei, G.; Lundmark, A.; Benchimol, D.; Lee, L.; Hu, Y.O.O.; Kats, A.; Saevarsdottir, S.; Catrina, A.I.; Klinge, B.; et al. Periodontal health and oral microbiota in patients with rheumatoid arthritis. *J. Clin. Med.* **2019**, *8*, 630. [CrossRef]
39. Fan, X.; Alekseyenko, A.V.; Wu, J.; Peters, B.A.; Jacobs, E.J.; Gapstur, S.M.; Purdue, M.P.; Abnet, C.C.; Stolzenberg-Solomon, R.; Miller, G.; et al. Human oral microbiome and prospective risk for pancreatic cancer: A population-based nested case-control study. *Gut* **2018**, *67*, 120–127. [CrossRef]
40. Han, Y.W. *Fusobacterium nucleatum*: A commensal-turned pathogen. *Curr. Opin. Microbiol.* **2015**, *23*, 141–147. [CrossRef]
41. Abed, J.; Maalouf, N.; Parhi, L.; Chaushu, S.; Mandelboim, O.; Bachrach, G. Tumor targeting by *Fusobacterium nucleatum*: A pilot study and future perspectives. *Front. Cell. Infect. Microbiol.* **2017**, *7*, 295. [CrossRef] [PubMed]
42. Gursoy, U.K.; Könönen, E.; Luukkonen, N.; Uitto, V.J. Human neutrophil defensins and their effect on epithelial cells. *J. Periodontol.* **2013**, *84*, 126–133. [CrossRef] [PubMed]
43. Benakanakere, M.; Kinane, D.F. Innate cellular responses to the periodontal biofilm. *Front. Oral Biol.* **2012**, *15*, 41–55. [PubMed]
44. Cekici, A.; Kantarci, A.; Hasturk, H.; Van Dyke, T.E. Inflammatory and immune pathways in the pathogenesis of periodontal disease. *Periodontol. 2000* **2014**, *64*, 57–80. [CrossRef] [PubMed]
45. Damgaard, C.; Holmstrup, P.; Van Dyke, T.E.; Nielsen, C.H. The complement system and its role in the pathogenesis of periodontitis: Current concepts. *J. Periodontal Res.* **2015**, *50*, 283–293. [CrossRef]
46. Liu, J.; Du, X.; Chen, J.; Hu, L.; Chen, L. The induction expression of human β-defensins in gingival epithelial cells and fibroblasts. *Arch. Oral Biol.* **2013**, *58*, 1415–1421. [CrossRef]
47. Kasnak, G.; Könönen, E.; Syrjänen, S.; Gürsoy, M.; Zeidán-Chuliá, F.; Firatli, E.; Gürsoy, U.K. NFE2L2/NRF2, OGG1, and cytokine responses of human gingival keratinocytes against oxidative insults of various origin. *Mol. Cell. Biochem.* **2019**, *452*, 63–70. [CrossRef]
48. Song, B.; Zhang, Y.L.; Chen, L.J.; Zhou, T.; Huang, W.K.; Zhou, X.; Shao, L.Q. The role of Toll-like receptors in periodontitis. *Oral Dis.* **2017**, *23*, 168–180. [CrossRef]
49. Elmanfi, S.; Zhou, J.; Sintim, H.O.; Könönen, E.; Gürsoy, M.; Gürsoy, U.K. Regulation of gingival epithelial cytokine response by bacterial cyclic dinucleotides. *J. Oral Microbiol.* **2018**, *11*, 1538927. [CrossRef]
50. Fteita, D.; Könönen, E.; Gürsoy, M.; Ma, X.; Sintim, H.O.; Gürsoy, U.K. Quorum sensing molecules regulate epithelial cytokine response and biofilm-related virulence of three *Prevotella* species. *Anaerobe* **2018**, *54*, 128–135. [CrossRef]
51. Hiroshima, Y.; Bando, M.; Kataoka, M.; Inagaki, Y.; Herzberg, M.C.; Ross, K.F.; Hosoi, K.; Nagata, T.; Kido, J. Regulation of antimicrobial peptide expression in human gingival keratinocytes by interleukin-1α. *Arch. Oral Biol.* **2011**, *56*, 761–767. [CrossRef] [PubMed]
52. Jura, J.; Skalniak, L.; Koj, A. Monocyte chemotactic protein-1-induced protein-1 (MCPIP1) is a novel multifunctional modulator of inflammatory reactions. *Biochim. Biophys. Acta* **2012**, *1823*, 1905–1913. [CrossRef] [PubMed]
53. Cavalla, F.; Hernández-Rios, P.; Sorsa, T.; Biguetti, C.; Hernández, M. Matrix metalloproteinases as regulators of periodontal inflammation. *Int. J. Mol. Sci.* **2017**, *18*, 440.
54. Wilensky, A.; Segev, H.; Mizraji, G.; Shaul, Y.; Capucha, T.; Shacham, M.; Hovav, A.H. Dendritic cells and their role in periodontal disease. *Oral Dis.* **2014**, *20*, 119–126. [CrossRef] [PubMed]

55. Song, L.; Dong, G.; Guo, L.; Graves, D.T. The function of dendritic cells in modulating the host response. *Mol. Oral Microbiol.* **2018**, *33*, 13–21. [CrossRef] [PubMed]
56. Cheng, W.C.; Hughes, F.J.; Taams, L.S. The presence, function and regulation of IL-17 and Th17 cells in periodontitis. *J. Clin. Periodontol.* **2014**, *41*, 541–549. [CrossRef] [PubMed]
57. Alnaeeli, M.; Penninger, J.M.; Teng, Y.T. Immune interactions with CD4+ T cells promote the development of functional osteoclasts from murine CD11c+ dendritic cells. *J. Immunol.* **2006**, *177*, 3314–3326. [CrossRef] [PubMed]
58. Parkos, C.A. Neutrophil-epithelial interactions: A double-edged sword. *Am. J. Pathol.* **2016**, *186*, 1404–1416. [CrossRef] [PubMed]
59. Fine, N.; Hassanpour, S.; Borenstein, A.; Sima, C.; Oveisi, M.; Scholey, J.; Cherney, D.; Glogauer, M. Distinct oral neutrophil subsets define health and periodontal disease states. *J. Dent. Res.* **2016**, *95*, 931–938. [CrossRef] [PubMed]
60. Hajishengallis, G.; Moutsopoulos, N.M.; Hajishengallis, E.; Chavakis, T. Immune and regulatory functions of neutrophils in inflammatory bone loss. *Semin. Immunol.* **2016**, *28*, 146–158. [CrossRef] [PubMed]
61. Matthews, J.B.; Wright, H.J.; Roberts, A.; Ling-Mountford, N.; Cooper, P.R.; Chapple, I.L. Neutrophil hyper-responsiveness in periodontitis. *J. Dent. Res.* **2007**, *86*, 718–722. [CrossRef] [PubMed]
62. Ling, M.R.; Chapple, I.L.; Matthews, J.B. Peripheral blood neutrophil cytokine hyper-reactivity in chronic periodontitis. *Innate Immun.* **2015**, *21*, 714–725. [CrossRef] [PubMed]
63. Olsen, I.; Hajishengallis, G. Major neutrophil functions subverted by *Porphyromonas gingivalis*. *J. Oral Microbiol.* **2016**, *8*, 30936. [CrossRef] [PubMed]
64. Sochalska, M.; Potempa, J. Manipulation of neutrophils by *Porphyromonas gingivalis* in the development of periodontitis. *Front. Cell. Infect. Microbiol.* **2017**, *7*, 197. [CrossRef] [PubMed]
65. Davies, L.C.; Rosas, M.; Jenkins, S.J.; Liao, C.T.; Scurr, M.J.; Brombacher, F.; Fraser, D.J.; Allen, J.E.; Jones, S.A.; Taylor, P.R. Distinct bone marrow-derived and tissue-resident macrophage lineages proliferate at key stages during inflammation. *Nat. Commun.* **2013**, *4*, 1886. [CrossRef] [PubMed]
66. Hajishengallis, G.; Sahingur, S.E. Novel inflammatory pathways in periodontitis. *Adv. Dent. Res.* **2014**, *26*, 23–29. [CrossRef] [PubMed]
67. Garlet, G.P.; Giannobile, W.V. Macrophages: The bridge between inflammation resolution and tissue repair? *J. Dent. Res.* **2018**, *97*, 1079–1081. [CrossRef] [PubMed]
68. Papadopoulos, G.; Shaik-Dasthagirisaheb, Y.B.; Huang, N.; Viglianti, G.A.; Henderson, A.J.; Kantarci, A.; Gibson, F.C. Immunologic environment influences macrophage response to *Porphyromonas gingivalis*. *Mol. Oral Microbiol.* **2017**, *32*, 250–261. [CrossRef] [PubMed]
69. Dutzan, N.; Konkel, J.E.; Greenwell-Wild, T.; Moutsopoulos, N.M. Characterization of the human immune cell network at the gingival barrier. *Mucosal Immunol.* **2016**, *9*, 1163–1172. [CrossRef] [PubMed]
70. Campbell, L.; Millhouse, E.; Malcolm, J.; Culshaw, S. T cells, teeth and tissue destruction - what do T cells do in periodontal disease? *Mol. Oral Microbiol.* **2016**, *31*, 445–456. [CrossRef] [PubMed]
71. Loos, B.G.; Papantonopoulos, G.; Jepsen, S.; Laine, M.L. What is the contribution of genetics to periodontal risk? *Dent. Clin. North Am.* **2015**, *59*, 761–780. [CrossRef]
72. Bosshardt, D.D.; Lang, N.P. The junctional epithelium: From health to disease. *J Dent. Res.* **2005**, *84*, 9–20. [CrossRef]
73. Lang, N.P.; Schätzle, M.A.; Löe, H. Gingivitis as a risk factor in periodontal disease. *J. Clin. Periodontol.* **2009**, *36* (Suppl. 10), 3–8. [CrossRef]
74. Henderson, B.; Kaiser, F. Bacterial modulators of bone remodeling in the periodontal pocket. *Periodontol. 2000* **2018**, *76*, 97–108. [CrossRef]
75. Sorsa, T.; Tjäderhane, L.; Konttinen, Y.T.; Lauhio, A.; Salo, T.; Lee, H.M.; Golub, L.M.; Brown, D.L.; Mäntylä, P. Matrix metalloproteinases: Contribution to pathogenesis, diagnosis and treatment of periodontal inflammation. *Ann. Med.* **2006**, *38*, 306–321. [CrossRef]
76. Kurgan, S.; Kantarci, A. Molecular basis for immunohistochemical and inflammatory changes during progression of gingivitis to periodontitis. *Periodontol. 2000* **2018**, *76*, 51–67. [CrossRef]
77. Belibasakis, G.N.; Bostanci, N. The RANKL-OPG system in clinical periodontology. *J. Clin. Periodontol.* **2012**, *39*, 239–248. [CrossRef]

78. Gursoy, U.K.; Könönen, E.; Huumonen, S.; Tervahartiala, T.; Pussinen, P.J.; Suominen, A.L.; Sorsa, T. Salivary type I collagen degradation end-products and related matrix metalloproteinases in periodontitis. *J. Clin. Periodontol.* **2013**, *40*, 18–25. [CrossRef]
79. Reynolds, M.A.; Kao, R.T.; Camargo, P.M.; Caton, J.G.; Clem, D.S.; Fiorellini, J.P.; Geisinger, M.L.; Mills, M.P.; Nares, S.; Nevins, M.L. Periodontal regeneration - intrabony defects: A consensus report from the AAP regeneration workshop. *J. Periodontol.* **2015**, *86* (Suppl. 2), 105–107. [CrossRef]
80. Bunaes, D.F.; Lie, S.A.; Enersen, M.; Aastrøm, A.N.; Mustafa, K.; Leknes, K.N. Site-specific treatment outcome in smokers following non-surgical and surgical periodontal therapy. *J. Clin. Periodontol.* **2015**, *42*, 933–942. [CrossRef]
81. Ryder, M.I.; Couch, E.T.; Chaffee, B.W. Personalized periodontal treatment for the tobacco- and alcohol-using patient. *Periodontol. 2000* **2018**, *78*, 30–46. [CrossRef]
82. Delima, S.L.; McBride, R.K.; Preshaw, P.M.; Heasman, P.A.; Kumar, P.S. Response of subgingival bacteria to smoking cessation. *J. Clin. Microbiol.* **2010**, *48*, 2344–2449. [CrossRef]
83. Haffajee, A.D.; Teles, R.P.; Socransky, S.S. The effect of periodontal therapy on the composition of the subgingival microbiota. *Periodontol* **2006**, *42*, 219–258. [CrossRef]
84. Axelsson, P.; Nyström, B.; Lindhe, J. The long-term effect of a plaque control program on tooth mortality, caries and periodontal disease in adults. Results after 30 years of maintenance. *J. Clin. Periodontol.* **2004**, *31*, 749–757. [CrossRef]
85. Rosling, B.; Serino, G.; Hellström, M.K.; Socransky, S.S.; Lindhe, J. Longitudinal periodontal tissue alterations during supportive therapy. Findings from subjects with normal and high susceptibility to periodontal disease. *J. Clin. Periodontol.* **2001**, *28*, 241–249. [CrossRef]
86. Müller, S.; Eickholz, P.; Reitmeir, P.; Eger, T. Long-term tooth loss in periodontally compromised but treated patients according to the type of prosthodontic treatment. A retrospective study. *J. Oral Rehabil.* **2013**, *40*, 358–367. [CrossRef]
87. Paraskevas, S.; Huizinga, J.D.; Loos, B.G. A systematic review and meta-analyses on C-reactive protein in relation to periodontitis. *J. Clin. Periodontol.* **2008**, *35*, 277–290. [CrossRef]
88. Tonetti, M.S.; D'Aiuto, F.; Nibali, L.; Donald, A.; Storry, C.; Parkar, M.; Suvan, J.; Hingorani, A.D.; Vallance, P.; Deanfield, J. Treatment of periodontitis and endothelial function. *N. Engl. J. Med.* **2007**, *356*, 911–920. [CrossRef]
89. Teeuw, W.J.; Slot, D.E.; Susanto, H.; Gerdes, V.E.; Abbas, F.; D'Aiuto, F.; Kastelein, J.J.; Loos, B.G.J. Treatment of periodontitis improves the atherosclerotic profile: A systematic review and meta-analysis. *J. Clin. Periodontol.* **2014**, *41*, 70–79. [CrossRef]
90. Wang, X.; Han, X.; Guo, X.; Luo, X.; Wang, D. The effect of periodontal treatment on hemoglobin A1c levels of diabetic patients: A systematic review and meta-analysis. *PLoS ONE* **2014**, *9*, e108412. [CrossRef]
91. D'Aiuto, F.; Gkranias, N.; Bhowruth, D.; Khan, T.; Orlandi, M.; Suvan, J.; Masi, S.; Tsakos, G.; Hurel, S.; Hingorani, A.D.; et al. Systemic effects of periodontitis treatment in patients with type 2 diabetes: A 12 month, single-centre, investigator-masked, randomised trial. *Lancet Diabetes Endocrinol.* **2018**, *6*, 954–965.
92. Morand, D.N.; Davideau, J.L.; Clauss, F.; Jessel, N.; Tenenbaum, H.; Huck, O. Cytokines during periodontal wound healing: Potential application for new therapeutic approach. *Oral Dis.* **2017**, *23*, 300–311. [CrossRef]
93. Alvarez, C.; Rojas, C.; Rojas, L.; Cafferata, E.A.; Monasterio, G.; Vernal, R. Regulatory T lymphocytes in periodontitis: A translational view. *Mediators Inflamm.* **2018**, *2018*, 7806912. [CrossRef]

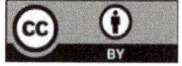

© 2019 by the authors. Licensee MDPI, Basel, Switzerland. This article is an open access article distributed under the terms and conditions of the Creative Commons Attribution (CC BY) license (http://creativecommons.org/licenses/by/4.0/).

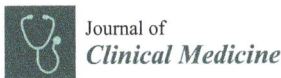

Review

Next Generation Sequencing Discoveries of the Nitrate-Responsive Oral Microbiome and Its Effect on Vascular Responses

Melissa M. Grant [1] and Daniel Jönsson [2,3,*]

1. School of Dentistry, Institute of Clinical Sciences, University of Birmingham and Birmingham Community Healthcare Foundation Trust, Birmingham B5 7EG, UK
2. Swedish Dental Service of Skåne, 222 37 Lund, Sweden
3. Department of Periodontology, Faculty of Odontology, Malmö University, 214 21 Malmö, Sweden
* Correspondence: daniel.jonsson@mau.se; Tel.: +46-406-658-553

Received: 30 June 2019; Accepted: 24 July 2019; Published: 26 July 2019

Abstract: Cardiovascular disease is a worldwide human condition which has multiple underlying contributing factors: one of these is long-term increased blood pressure—hypertension. Nitric oxide (NO) is a small nitrogenous radical species that has a number of physiological functions including vasodilation. It can be produced enzymatically through host nitric oxide synthases and by an alternative nitrate–nitrite–NO pathway from ingested inorganic nitrate. It was discovered that this route relies on the ability of the oral microbiota to reduce nitrate to nitrite and NO. Next generation sequencing has been used over the past two decades to gain deeper insight into the microbes involved, their location and the effect of their removal from the oral cavity. This review article presents this research and comments briefly on future directions.

Keywords: oral microbiome; saliva; nitric oxide; nitrate; nitrite

1. Introduction

Oral microbiota are the second most complex niche of the human microbiome [1]; they have been associated with several non-communicative diseases, including cancer [2], Alzheimer's disease [3] and cardiovascular disease (CVD) [4,5]. The current review will focus on the association between the oral microbiota and the most well established mechanistic pathway through which the oral microbiota may modify CVD, namely via the nitric oxide (NO) synthesis pathway.

In Europe, 3.9 million people die yearly from CVD, costing about 210 billion Euros per year in healthcare costs, productivity losses and informal care [6]. Hypertension is an important subclinical parameter for cardiovascular disease—about 54% of all stroke and 47% of ischemic heart disease are attributed to hypertension [7]. Hypertension is defined by WHO as systolic blood pressure ≥140 mm Hg and diastolic pressure ≥90, however it was recently reported that the definition of hypertension needs to be re-visited as lowering systolic blood pressure not to under 140 mm Hg, but to 120 mm Hg causes less fatal and non-fatal cardiovascular events. This also suggests that hypertension may be more important in CVD than previously described [8].

There are several important mechanisms behind hypertension, but one key underpinning is the L-arginine/NO synthesis pathway. In addition to hypertension, the NO synthesis pathway is important in the pathobiology of CVD via inflammation and platelet activation and aggregation [9].

2. The L-Arginine/NO Synthesis Pathway

In 1998, Robert F. Furchgott, Louis J. Ignarro and Ferid Murad were awarded the Nobel Prize for detecting and describing L-arginine/NO synthesis in cardiovascular physiology and disease. Furchgott described the accidental finding that acetylcholine, bradykinin, histamine and 5-hydroxytryptamine relax isolated preparations of blood vessels, but only when the endothelium is intact. In rabbit thoracic aorta prepared as a transverse ring, acetylcholine stimulation with muscarinic agonists caused dilatation, but not in aorta prepared as a helical strip. Later, it was noted that gently rubbing the endothelium of the transverse ring preparations similarly caused loss of smooth muscle cell relaxation. The endothelium-derived factor relaxing the smooth muscle cells lining the arteries was named endothelium-derived relaxing factor (EDRF) [10,11].

Following the discovery of EDRF, there was a wave of research inhibiting EDRF. What these inhibitors all had in common was their redox potency, except hemoglobin which inactivated EDRF by binding to it. This led to the suggestion that EDRF might be a free radical [12,13], and eventually Ignarro et al. [14] suggested that EDRF may in fact be NO, which at that time was not known to be synthesized in humans.

Then the question was where NO originates from, and in macrophages it was shown that NO originates from L-arginine [15,16]. Later, the enzyme responsible for the conversion of L-arginine to NO was identified as NO synthase. In addition to macrophages, NO was discovered in the central nervous system [17]. Depending on the system, different isoforms of NO synthase were identified, namely eNOS in endothelial cells, nNOS in the nervous system, and iNOS in the inflammatory system.

The inhibition of L-arginine and knockdown of eNOS in animal models led to the paradigm shift that hypertension is not due to increased resistance, but due to decreased conductance in the vascular system. The eNOS knockout mice also had increased endothelial-leucocyte interaction, platelet aggregation and thrombosis [18]. When knocking down eNOS in hypercholesterolemic ApoE mice, the eNOS-deficient mice had accelerated atherosclerosis [19]. Taken together, this work showed that the importance of eNOS and the L-arginine/NO synthesis pathway goes far beyond hypertension. In fact, NO from the eNOS activity of endothelial cells not only causes less contractility of the smooth muscle cells, but also results in inhibition of activation, adhesion and aggregation of platelets, less adhesivity of leucocytes and enhanced oxygen delivery from erythrocytes [20].

In 1986, Ludmer and coworkers [21] published a now classical study showing that in subjects with known CVD, acetylcholine resulted in a paradoxical NO-mediated vasoconstriction, in contrast to vasodilation in healthy subjects. Importantly, subjects with minimal CVD (angiographically) also displayed vasoconstriction. All three groups dilated in response to nitroglycerine. What this study suggested was that dysfunctional endothelial NO production and availability might precede the formation of clinically significant atherosclerotic lesions—today known as endothelial dysfunction. The clinical evaluation of endothelial function is through flow-mediated dilatation (FMD), today known as a subclinical predictor of CVD events [22] which is impaired in known CVD high risk groups, such as smokers and subjects with hypocholesteremia [23].

Endothelial dysfunction affects the L-arginine/NO-synthesis in two important ways—on a cellular level and on a molecular level. Endothelial cells can undergo phenotypical changes from healthy to a pro-inflammatory cell type. Healthy conditions, such as laminar blood flow, cause upregulation of transcription factors, such as Kruppel-like factors (KLF) 2 and 4, whereas athero-promoting flow and pro-inflammatory content of the blood cause upregulation of NFkB, eliciting a pro-inflammatory cell phenotype [24,25]. KLF2 promotes anti-CVD mechanisms, such as anti-inflammation by inhibiting the NFkB pathway [26,27], and anti-thrombogenic by inducing eNOS and thrombomodulin and reducing plasminogen activator inhibitor (PAI-1) [28]. Interestingly, KLF2 can be induced pharmacologically, via statins that exert atheroprotective effects via KLF2 [29]. NFkB is a pro-inflammatory transcription factor causing recruitment and activation of leucocytes at the site and subsequent endothelial dysfunction [24,25]. On a molecular level, the inflammatory micro-environment at an atherosclerotic lesion causes a net excess of reactive oxygen species (ROS), including superoxide which inactivates NO by forming peroxynitrite which could result in DNA damage and protein modification, but also through uncoupling of eNOS [30].

3. Microbiome Contributions to NO Synthesis

Research in the mid-1990s showed that NO production can be independent of NOS [31–33]. This production was linked directly to diet as, for example, nitrate-rich vegetable consumption could increase systemic nitrate and result in lowering of systolic blood pressure [34]. However, the activation of nitrate and transformation ultimately to NO requires its conversion to nitrite and mammals lack the enzymes required for this bioactivation. Termed the entero-salivary circulation, this requires consumption of nitrate which is absorbed by the upper gastrointestinal tract (Figure 1). Nitrate in circulation (approximately 25%, the remainder being secreted by the kidneys) is then selectively acquired by the sialin protein in the salivary glands and thus a high concentration of nitrate (1500 µM) is returned to the oral cavity [35]. There, the conversion of nitrate to nitrite is carried out by the oral microbiota [36]. Upon entering the stomach, the nitrite is protonated to nitrous acid (HNO_2) which can then decompose to NO and other oxides. The following section reviews the results from next generation sequencing approaches to understanding more about the bacteria involved in the conversion of nitrate to nitrite in the oral cavity.

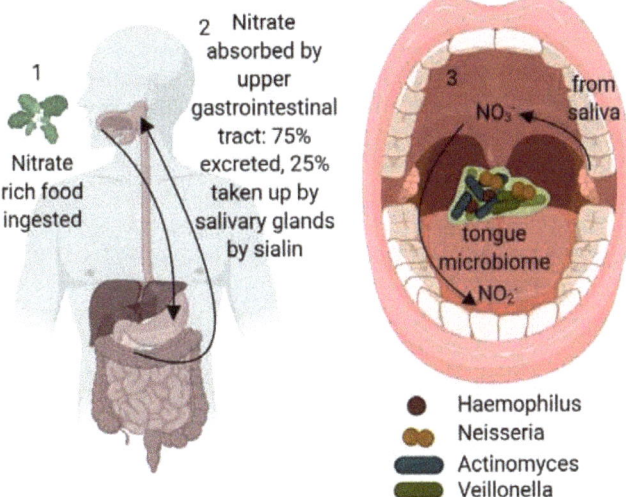

Figure 1. Enterosalivary nitrate production and the role of the oral microbiome. 1. Nitrate-rich food, such as leafy green vegetables, is ingested. 2. Nitrate is absorbed in the upper gastrointestinal tract and 25% is then found in saliva due to the action of the sialin anion transporter. 3. The oral microflora, particularly nitrate-reducing bacteria, such as *Actinomyces, Haemophilus, Neisseria* and *Veillonella*, residing in the dorsal tongue biofilm convert nitrate to nitrite, and also to nitric oxide (NO) which can be absorbed through the vascularized tongue or through swallowing back in to the gastrointestinal system for absorption. Image created in Biorender.

The first study examining the oral microbiota and the constituent microbes involved in nitrate and nitrite reduction was published in 2005 [36]. By mapping nitrate reduction across the mouth, Doel et al. could demonstrate that the majority of nitrate reductase activity was associated with the dorsum of the tongue. Indeed, the tongue dorsum has a distinct microbiome which is related to the other oral niches. It is more similar to the saliva microbiome than to the oral plaque microbiomes (Human microbiome project consortium 2012 [37]). They went further by isolating and culturing species associated within this site and verifying nitrate reductase activity. More species were found to have this activity under anaerobic conditions than aerobic conditions. Isolates of interest were 16S rRNA sequenced to gain their identity. The highest levels of nitrate reduction were found with

Actinomyces odontolytica which was the second most common tongue isolate, though the authors also detected *Veillonella atypica, Veillonella dispar, Veillonella parvula, Actinomyces naeslundii, Actinomyces viscosus, Rothia dentocariosa, Rothia mucilaginosa, Staphylococcus epidermidis, Staphylococcus hemolyticus, Corynebacterium matruchotii, Corynebacterium durum, Haemophilus parainfluenzae, Haemophilus segnis, Propionibacterium acnes, Granulicatella adiacens, Selenomonas noxia, Capnocytophaga sputigena, Eikinella corrodens* and *Microbacterium oxydans*. The next report showing the microbiome associated with nitrate reduction was published a decade later, once the metagenomics analysis tools had matured more fully. Hyde et al. [4] used 16S rRNA and whole genome analysis of whole tongue scrapings and of biofilms originated from the scrapings matured on polymethacrylate (PMMA) discs for up to 4 days. The change in technique from Doel et al. [36] allowed for a larger number of operational taxonomic units (OTUs) to be discovered and a wider range of genera: *Streptococcus, Veillonella, Prevotella, Neisseria* and *Haemophilus*. The authors noted that there was a wide variation between different donors. With the samples that were used to inoculate biofilms, it was also noted that the number of OTUs dropped dramatically within the first 24 h and that by 4 days the biofilms were dominated by the *Streptococcal* species. Koopman et al. [38] also demonstrated this loss of diversity when growing saliva samples in a nitrate-reducing bacteria discovery study. This is of interest in light of the report by Doel et al. where culturing was used to find the nitrate-reducing bacteria before sequencing as this may have resulted in under-estimation of the discoveries. With the whole genome sequencing and pathway analysis, by Hyde et al., the pathways associated with the samples were more consistent with a match across the top eight pathways, such as various amino acid metabolic or synthetic pathways and nitrogen metabolism. Hyde et al. also split their results into samples with high, intermediate and low nitrate reductase activity: these samples were derived from the inoculated biofilms and were derived from individual donors creating a dataset of 30. Using principal coordinate analysis (PCoA), they showed that the samples with high nitrate reduction capacity were more likely to contain *Granulicatella, Veillonella, Neisseria, Actinomyces, Prevotella, Haemophilus, Fusobacterium* and some unclassified species of the *Gemellaceae* family. Some of these were already known whilst others were novel. Of note was the fact that *Lactobacillus* was associated with the least nitrate-reducing samples and the authors speculated that these genera may have an inhibitory role through production of some unknown byproduct that may inhibit nitrate reduction in those communities. Last, these authors also grew four microorganisms with putative nitrate and/or nitrite reduction capacity: *A. odontolyticus, V. dispar, F. nucleatum* and *S. mutans*. This last aspect of their study showed that these species could work independently or in a consortium to effectively remove nitrate and/or nitrite from growth medium. This is an important illustration of the complex interdependent networks in which biofilms exist. This paper not only confirmed previous findings but took them a step further, however both studies relied on discoveries from only 10 and 6 tongue scraping donors.

Hyde et al. [39] also published an article characterizing the tongue microbiome of rats, in comparison to human tongue scrapings, with a focus on the effect of dietary nitrate. One of the main findings was that the rat tongue microbiome was less diverse and appeared to be missing or had a greatly decreased amount of *Veillonella, Prevotella, Neisseria* and *Porphyromonas* in comparison to human samples. However, one of the limitations of the study was that different methodologies were used between the rat and human samples. Nevertheless, they could also examine the effect of administration of sodium nitrate via drinking water and chlorhexidine via oral rinse. The supplementation by sodium nitrate significantly decreased diastolic blood pressure and heart rate and made non-significant decreases in systolic blood pressure and mean arterial pressure. These changes were associated with relative increases in tongue *Haemophilus* species and *Streptococcus* species, which are nitrate and nitrite reducers, respectively. The change in the microbiome had not previously been demonstrated but later Koopman et al. [38] used a saliva inoculum from two human donors to create microcosms in the multiplaque artificial mouth (MAM) biofilm model system and to examine the effect of nitrate supplementation on the resultant microcosms. For one donor, *Neisseria* were associated with the nitrate-treated microcosms whereas *Veillonella* was more associated with nitrate treatment in the microcosms from the other donor. As both these genera seem to be missing from the rat tongue microbiome and this human study used saliva, it is difficult to draw a conclusion from a comparison of these experiments.

Chlorhexidine can abolish the effect of sodium nitrate supplementation [34,40–42] and Hyde et al. [39,43] showed that its use as a mouth rinse in rats decreased *Haemophilus, Aggregaterbacter,* and *Micrococcaceae* but increased *Enterobacteriaceae, Corynebacterium* and *Morganella* with the overall effect being an increase in diversity through a change in low abundance taxa in the baseline samples. Unfortunately, the chlorhexidine oral rinse did not change the blood pressure or heart rate measures as expected and the authors concluded that it did not remain in the mouth for long enough to exert the intended effect.

Recently, attention has turned towards responses in a wider range of donors. Vanhatalo et al. [43] examined the oral microbiome in young and old healthy donors and the response of these microbiomes to supplementation using a crossover design with either a high nitrate beetroot drink or placebo nitrate depleted over 10 days each. The supplementation of the high nitrate beetroot juice increased plasma nitrate to a similar extent whereas nitrite increases were greater for older participants. Mean arterial pressure, systolic blood pressure and diastolic blood pressure all showed a greater decrease with age and nitrite dose. Overall, they showed high quantities of *Fusobacterium nucleatum nucleatum, Prevotella melaninogenica, Campylobacter concisus, Leptotrichia buccalis, Veillonella parvula, Prevotella intermedia, Fusobacterium nucleatum vincentii* and *Neisseria meningitidis* in the tongue swabs. Changes in the oral microbiome were assessed in saliva samples before and after nitrate supplementation: supplementation changed the oral microbial communities but age did not and diversity was similar across the categories. Fifty-two taxonomic units were significantly changed with supplementation: *Veillonella* and *Prevotella* decreased, whereas *Neisseria* increased and there was no observed change in *Campylobacter* or *Haemophilus*. Burleigh et al. [44] studied the effect of nitrate-rich beetroot juice or nitrate-depleted placebo supplementation on the tongue microbiome and how the altered microbiome responded to an acute dose of nitrate. As seen before, there were decreases in *Prevotella, Streptococcus* and *Actinomyces* and an increase in *Neisseria* with supplementation. For the acute dose, saliva and plasma nitrate and nitrite were measured 1.5 h and 2.5 h, respectively, after nitrate consumption both before and after 7 days of supplementation. At both time points, there was an increase in nitrate and nitrite in both compartments but the alteration of the microbiome by 7 days of beetroot juice consumption did not alter the maximal nitrite and nitrate concentrations after the acute dose. The authors suggest that excess nitrite may be rapidly excreted to prevent excessive drops in blood pressure, or that the change in the nitrate/nitrite-reducing genera (*Prevotella* and *Actinomyces*) may balance the overall capacity of the system.

Kapil et al. [45] explored the influence of gender on nitrate reduction and the oral microbiota. Female participants had higher saliva, plasma and urine nitrite levels than males, and after supplementation with inorganic nitrate they showed a greater increase in plasma nitrate. However, there was no difference between the composition of the salivary microbiota of male and female participants. Ashworth et al. [46] considered the difference in the oral microbiome and dietary intake of inorganic nitrate between vegetarians and omnivores, as previously it was suggested that vegetarian diets are associated with lower blood pressure [47] and this is associated with higher nitrate intake [48]. By using dietary questionnaires, they demonstrated no difference in the consumption of nitrate and that saliva and plasma levels of nitrate and nitrite were similar between the two groups. The oral microbiome was similar between the two groups. The authors also administered a chlorhexidine mouth rinse intervention for 7 days and this caused a decrease in diversity in both groups and a drop in nitrate-reducing bacteria in both groups. Thus, this study suggested no differences in macrodiet and oral microbiome. This is in contrast to previous studies [49–51] which could be due to differences in the individuals examined across studies.

Tribble et al. [52] described the effect of tongue cleaning on the tongue microbiome and nitrate levels. Tongue cleaning is a technique that has been used for the removal of oral malodor or halitosis that is often ascribed to the tongue coating [53]. In this study, orally and systemically healthy oral health professionals were followed over the course of eleven days during which samples (tongue scrapings and saliva) were taken at baseline, at 7 days after use of the chlorhexidine mouth rinse and after a further 3 and 7 days after recovery from use of the mouth rinse. Chlorhexidine caused an increase in systolic blood pressure in the range of 5 mm/Hg which is equivalent to manipulation of dietary salt intake [54], however the donors were also stratified by the frequency of tongue cleaning as either none, once or twice per day. For those participants cleaning their tongue twice per day, there was the greatest increase in systolic blood pressure after the use of chlorhexidine. When examining the tongue microflora, the most common operational taxonomic unit was *Haemophilus parainfluenzae* and the second *Neisseria subflava*. However, the most common genus changed between individuals with groups of *Neisseria*, *Prevotella* and *Leptotrichia* as the most common. The frequency of tongue cleaning changed the abundance of species found: for example, *Leptotrichia spp* were detected in higher abundance on tongues that were not cleaned and daily cleaning (either once or twice) increased the abundance of *H. parainfluenzae* found. This showed that the tongue microbiome when tongue cleaning was implemented has a greater nitrate reductase capability. However, chlorhexidine treatment did not cause large-scale changes in the microbiome community. Further exploration suggested that any changes that occur are transient, with the recovery phase being associated with an increase in bacterial metabolic activity.

Box 1: Definitions:

- 16S rRNA is part of the bacterial ribosome, assigning structural scaffolding, and is of interest in the phylogenetic assignment of bacteria due to its slow rate of evolution.
- OTUs (operational taxonomic units) group together closely related individuals when individuals cannot be distinguished by the data available.
- Biofilms are embedded collections of microorganisms growing together in a matrix of extracellular polymeric substances on a surface.
- Next generation sequencing describes a wide range of DNA sequencing technologies capable of sequencing millions of fragments of DNA in parallel.
- Whole genome analysis sequences the whole of one or more genomes rather than a single gene, as with 16S rRNA analysis.
- Microbiome defines all of the microbial genomes in a given sample or environment.
- Microbiota defines the entire microbial flora in a given sample or environment.
- Principal coordinate analysis (PCoA) is a multivariate statistical technique used to reduce dimensions in data analysis and allowed for representation of the data visually.

4. Concluding Remarks

Overall, these next generation sequencing studies have demonstrated that there are nitrate and nitrite-reducing bacteria found in the mouth and that their removal through mouth rinsing with chlorhexidine will cause a temporary increase in blood pressure. The microbes most often found in the studies were from *Actinomyces*, *Haemophilus*, *Neisseria* and *Veillonella* genera. Samples have been from the tongue dorsum, where nitrate-reducing species were first identified, and also in saliva which may be easier to collect. The microbiomes of these two compartments are distinct but closely related. Furthermore, saliva indeed bathes the tongue, thereby enabling that microbiome to be sampled. More recent studies are just beginning to report [43–46,52] on how the microbiota in both the tongue dorsum and saliva change with different conditions, as previously only samples from homogeneous and healthy donors have been described. The number of donors in each study is also rising, helped by decreases in the costs of these types of experiments, which will help to gain more generalizable data and data that may reveal more subtle nuances between diseases types, ethnicities and other characteristics. This review has highlighted the role of the oral microbiota in the conversion of nitrate to nitrite and its importance to systemic balance. Understanding more about the role that the oral microbiota can play will enable future interventions that may aid with a stratified medicine approach that may rely more on bolstering the useful oral microflora and potentially reduce the use of antimicrobials.

Author Contributions: M.M.G. and D.J. Writing—Original draft, review and editing.

Funding: Daniel Jönsson's research time is sponsored by Swedish Dental Service of Skåne and Oral Health Related Research by Region Skåne.

Conflicts of Interest: The authors declare no conflict of interest.

References

1. Deo, P.N.; Deshmukh, R. Oral microbiome: Unveiling the fundamentals. *J. Oral Maxillofac. Pathol.* **2019**, *23*, 122–128. [PubMed]
2. Chen, J.; Domingue, J.C.; Sears, C.L. Microbiota dysbiosis in select human cancers: Evidence of association and causality. *Semin. Immunol.* **2017**, *32*, 25–34. [CrossRef] [PubMed]
3. Dominy, S.S.; Lynch, C.; Ermini, F.; Benedyk, M.; Marczyk, A.; Konradi, A.; Nguyen, M.; Haditsch, U.; Raha, D.; Griffin, C.; et al. Porphyromonas gingivalis in Alzheimer's disease brains: Evidence for disease causation and treatment with small-molecule inhibitors. *Sci. Adv.* **2019**, *5*, eaau3333. [CrossRef] [PubMed]
4. Hyde, E.R.; Andrade, F.; Vaksman, Z.; Parthasarathy, K.; Jiang, H.; Parthasarathy, D.K.; Torregrossa, A.C.; Tribble, G.; Kaplan, H.B.; Petrosino, J.F.; et al. Metagenomic analysis of nitrate-reducing bacteria in the oral cavity: Implications for nitric oxide homeostasis. *PLoS ONE* **2014**, *9*, e88645. [CrossRef] [PubMed]
5. Desvarieux, M.; Demmer, R.T.; Rundek, T.; Boden-Albala, B.; Jacobs, D.R., Jr.; Sacco, R.L.; Papapanou, P.N. Periodontal microbiota and carotid intima-media thickness: The Oral Infections and Vascular Disease Epidemiology Study (INVEST). *Circulation* **2005**, *111*, 576–582. [CrossRef] [PubMed]
6. Timmis, A.; Townsend, N.; Gale, C.; Grobbee, R.; Maniadakis, N.; Flather, M.; Wilkins, E.; Wright, L.; Vos, R.; Bax, J.; et al. European Society of Cardiology: Cardiovascular Disease Statistics 2017. *Eur. Heart J.* **2018**, *39*, 508–579. [CrossRef]
7. Lawes, C.M.; Vander Hoorn, S.; Rodgers, A.; for the International Society of Hypertension. Global burden of blood-pressure-related disease, 2001. *Lancet* **2008**, *371*, 1513–1518. [CrossRef]
8. Group, S.R.; Wright, J.T., Jr.; Williamson, J.D.; Whelton, P.K.; Snyder, J.K.; Sink, K.M.; Rocco, M.V.; Reboussin, D.M.; Rahman, M.; Oparil, S.; et al. A Randomized Trial of Intensive versus Standard Blood-Pressure Control. *N. Engl. J. Med.* **2015**, *373*, 2103–2116. [CrossRef]
9. Radomski, M.W.; Palmer, R.M.; Moncada, S. An L-arginine/nitric oxide pathway present in human platelets regulates aggregation. *Proc. Natl. Acad. Sci. USA* **1990**, *87*, 5193–5197. [CrossRef]
10. Furchgott, R.F. The 1996 Albert Lasker Medical Research Awards. The discovery of endothelium-derived relaxing factor and its importance in the identification of nitric oxide. *JAMA* **1996**, *276*, 1186–1188. [CrossRef]
11. Furchgott, R.F.; Zawadzki, J.V. The obligatory role of endothelial cells in the relaxation of arterial smooth muscle by acetylcholine. *Nature* **1980**, *288*, 373–376. [CrossRef] [PubMed]
12. Gryglewski, R.J.; Palmer, R.M.; Moncada, S. Superoxide anion is involved in the breakdown of endothelium-derived vascular relaxing factor. *Nature* **1986**, *320*, 454–456. [CrossRef] [PubMed]
13. Moncada, S.; Palmer, R.M.; Gryglewski, R.J. Mechanism of action of some inhibitors of endothelium-derived relaxing factor. *Proc. Natl. Acad. Sci. USA* **1986**, *83*, 9164–9168. [CrossRef] [PubMed]
14. Ignarro, L.J.; Buga, G.M.; Wood, K.S.; Byrns, R.E.; Chaudhuri, G. Endothelium-derived relaxing factor produced and released from artery and vein is nitric oxide. *Proc. Natl. Acad. Sci. USA* **1987**, *84*, 9265–9269. [CrossRef] [PubMed]
15. Hibbs, J.B., Jr.; Taintor, R.R.; Vavrin, Z. Macrophage cytotoxicity: Role for L-arginine deiminase and imino nitrogen oxidation to nitrite. *Science* **1987**, *235*, 473–476. [CrossRef] [PubMed]
16. Iyengar, R.; Stuehr, D.J.; Marletta, M.A. Macrophage synthesis of nitrite, nitrate, and N-nitrosamines: Precursors and role of the respiratory burst. *Proc. Natl. Acad. Sci. USA* **1987**, *84*, 6369–6373. [CrossRef]
17. Moncada, S.; Palmer, R.M.; Higgs, E.A. Nitric oxide: Physiology, pathophysiology, and pharmacology. *Pharmacol. Rev.* **1991**, *43*, 109–142.
18. Moncada, S.; Higgs, E.A. The discovery of nitric oxide and its role in vascular biology. *Br. J. Pharmacol.* **2006**, *147* (Suppl. 1), S193–S201. [CrossRef]

19. Kuhlencordt, P.J.; Gyurko, R.; Han, F.; Scherrer-Crosbie, M.; Aretz, T.H.; Hajjar, R.; Picard, M.H.; Huang, P.L. Accelerated atherosclerosis, aortic aneurysm formation, and ischemic heart disease in apolipoprotein E/endothelial nitric oxide synthase double-knockout mice. *Circulation* **2001**, *104*, 448–454. [CrossRef]
20. Gimbrone, M.A., Jr.; Garcia-Cardena, G. Endothelial Cell Dysfunction and the Pathobiology of Atherosclerosis. *Circ. Res.* **2016**, *118*, 620–636. [CrossRef]
21. Ludmer, P.L.; Selwyn, A.P.; Shook, T.L.; Wayne, R.R.; Mudge, G.H.; Alexander, R.W.; Ganz, P. Paradoxical vasoconstriction induced by acetylcholine in atherosclerotic coronary arteries. *N. Engl. J. Med.* **1986**, *315*, 1046–1051. [CrossRef] [PubMed]
22. Yeboah, J.; Crouse, J.R.; Hsu, F.C.; Burke, G.L.; Herrington, D.M. Brachial flow-mediated dilation predicts incident cardiovascular events in older adults: The Cardiovascular Health Study. *Circulation* **2007**, *115*, 2390–2397. [CrossRef] [PubMed]
23. Celermajer, D.S.; Sorensen, K.E.; Gooch, V.M.; Spiegelhalter, D.J.; Miller, O.I.; Sullivan, I.D.; Lloyd, J.K.; Deanfield, J.E. Non-invasive detection of endothelial dysfunction in children and adults at risk of atherosclerosis. *Lancet* **1992**, *340*, 1111–1115. [CrossRef]
24. Atkins, G.B.; Simon, D.I. Interplay between NF-kappaB and Kruppel-like factors in vascular inflammation and atherosclerosis: Location, location, location. *J. Am. Heart Assoc.* **2013**, *2*, e000290. [CrossRef] [PubMed]
25. Davies, P.F.; Civelek, M.; Fang, Y.; Fleming, I. The atherosusceptible endothelium: Endothelial phenotypes in complex haemodynamic shear stress regions in vivo. *Cardiovasc. Res.* **2013**, *99*, 315–327. [CrossRef]
26. SenBanerjee, S.; Lin, Z.; Atkins, G.B.; Greif, D.M.; Rao, R.M.; Kumar, A.; Feinberg, M.W.; Chen, Z.; Simon, D.I.; Luscinskas, F.W.; et al. KLF2 Is a novel transcriptional regulator of endothelial proinflammatory activation. *J. Exp. Med.* **2004**, *199*, 1305–1315. [CrossRef]
27. Hamik, A.; Lin, Z.; Kumar, A.; Balcells, M.; Sinha, S.; Katz, J.; Feinberg, M.W.; Gerzsten, R.E.; Edelman, E.R.; Jain, M.K. Kruppel-like factor 4 regulates endothelial inflammation. *J. Biol. Chem.* **2007**, *282*, 13769–13779. [CrossRef]
28. Lin, Z.; Kumar, A.; SenBanerjee, S.; Staniszewski, K.; Parmar, K.; Vaughan, D.E.; Gimbrone, M.A., Jr.; Balasubramanian, V.; Garcia-Cardena, G.; Jain, M.K. Kruppel-like factor 2 (KLF2) regulates endothelial thrombotic function. *Circ. Res.* **2005**, *96*, e48–e57. [CrossRef]
29. Parmar, K.M.; Nambudiri, V.; Dai, G.; Larman, H.B.; Gimbrone, M.A., Jr.; Garcia-Cardena, G. Statins exert endothelial atheroprotective effects via the KLF2 transcription factor. *J. Biol. Chem.* **2005**, *280*, 26714–26719. [CrossRef]
30. Forstermann, U.; Xia, N.; Li, H. Roles of Vascular Oxidative Stress and Nitric Oxide in the Pathogenesis of Atherosclerosis. *Circ. Res.* **2017**, *120*, 713–735. [CrossRef]
31. Benjamin, N.; O'Driscoll, F.; Dougall, H.; Duncan, C.; Smith, L.; Golden, M.; McKenzie, H. Stomach NO synthesis. *Nature* **1994**, *368*, 502. [CrossRef] [PubMed]
32. Lundberg, J.O.; Weitzberg, E.; Lundberg, J.M.; Alving, K. Intragastric nitric oxide production in humans: Measurements in expelled air. *Gut* **1994**, *35*, 1543–1546. [CrossRef] [PubMed]
33. Zweier, J.L.; Wang, P.; Samouilov, A.; Kuppusamy, P. Enzyme-independent formation of nitric oxide in biological tissues. *Nat. Med.* **1995**, *1*, 804–809. [CrossRef] [PubMed]
34. Webb, A.J.; Patel, N.; Loukogeorgakis, S.; Okorie, M.; Aboud, Z.; Misra, S.; Rashid, R.; Miall, P.; Deanfield, J.; Benjamin, N.; et al. Acute blood pressure lowering, vasoprotective, and antiplatelet properties of dietary nitrate via bioconversion to nitrite. *Hypertension* **2008**, *51*, 784–790. [CrossRef] [PubMed]
35. Reimer, R.J. SLC17: A functionally diverse family of organic anion transporters. *Mol. Aspects Med.* **2013**, *34*, 350–359. [CrossRef] [PubMed]
36. Doel, J.J.; Benjamin, N.; Hector, M.P.; Rogers, M.; Allaker, R.P. Evaluation of bacterial nitrate reduction in the human oral cavity. *Eur. J. Oral Sci.* **2005**, *113*, 14–19. [CrossRef]
37. The Human Microbiome Project Consortium. Structure, function and diversity of the healthy human microbiome. *Nature* **2012**, *486*, 207–214. [CrossRef]
38. Koopman, J.E.; Buijs, M.J.; Brandt, B.W.; Keijser, B.J.; Crielaard, W.; Zaura, E. Nitrate and the Origin of Saliva Influence Composition and Short Chain Fatty Acid Production of Oral Microcosms. *Microb. Ecol.* **2016**, *72*, 479–492. [CrossRef]
39. Hyde, E.R.; Luk, B.; Cron, S.; Kusic, L.; McCue, T.; Bauch, T.; Kaplan, H.; Tribble, G.; Petrosino, J.F.; Bryan, N.S. Characterization of the rat oral microbiome and the effects of dietary nitrate. *Free Radic. Biol. Med.* **2014**, *77*, 249–257. [CrossRef]

40. Kapil, V.; Haydar, S.M.; Pearl, V.; Lundberg, J.O.; Weitzberg, E.; Ahluwalia, A. Physiological role for nitrate-reducing oral bacteria in blood pressure control. *Free Radic. Biol. Med.* **2013**, *55*, 93–100. [CrossRef]
41. Bondonno, C.P.; Liu, A.H.; Croft, K.D.; Considine, M.J.; Puddey, I.B.; Woodman, R.J.; Hodgson, J.M. Antibacterial mouthwash blunts oral nitrate reduction and increases blood pressure in treated hypertensive men and women. *Am. J. Hypertens.* **2015**, *28*, 572–575. [CrossRef] [PubMed]
42. Govoni, M.; Jansson, E.A.; Weitzberg, E.; Lundberg, J.O. The increase in plasma nitrite after a dietary nitrate load is markedly attenuated by an antibacterial mouthwash. *Nitric Oxide* **2008**, *19*, 333–337. [CrossRef] [PubMed]
43. Vanhatalo, A.; Blackwell, J.R.; L'Heureux, J.E.; Williams, D.W.; Smith, A.; van der Giezen, M.; Winyard, P.G.; Kelly, J.; Jones, A.M. Nitrate-responsive oral microbiome modulates nitric oxide homeostasis and blood pressure in humans. *Free Radic. Biol. Med.* **2018**, *124*, 21–30. [CrossRef] [PubMed]
44. Burleigh, M.; Liddle, L.; Muggeridge, D.J.; Monaghan, C.; Sculthorpe, N.; Butcher, J.; Henriquez, F.; Easton, C. Dietary nitrate supplementation alters the oral microbiome but does not improve the vascular responses to an acute nitrate dose. *Nitric Oxide* **2019**, *89*, 54–63. [CrossRef] [PubMed]
45. Kapil, V.; Rathod, K.S.; Khambata, R.S.; Bahra, M.; Velmurugan, S.; Purba, A.; Watson, D.S.; Barnes, M.R.; Wade, W.G.; Ahluwalia, A. Sex differences in the nitrate-nitrite-NO(*) pathway: Role of oral nitrate-reducing bacteria. *Free Radic. Biol. Med.* **2018**, *126*, 113–121. [CrossRef] [PubMed]
46. Ashworth, A.; Cutler, C.; Farnham, G.; Liddle, L.; Burleigh, M.; Rodiles, A.; Sillitti, C.; Kiernan, M.; Moore, M.; Hickson, M.; et al. Dietary intake of inorganic nitrate in vegetarians and omnivores and its impact on blood pressure, resting metabolic rate and the oral microbiome. *Free Radic. Biol. Med.* **2019**, *138*, 63–72. [CrossRef] [PubMed]
47. Yokoyama, Y.; Nishimura, K.; Barnard, N.D.; Takegami, M.; Watanabe, M.; Sekikawa, A.; Okamura, T.; Miyamoto, Y. Vegetarian diets and blood pressure: A meta-analysis. *JAMA Intern. Med.* **2014**, *174*, 577–587. [CrossRef]
48. Hord, N.G.; Tang, Y.; Bryan, N.S. Food sources of nitrates and nitrites: The physiologic context for potential health benefits. *Am. J. Clin. Nutr.* **2009**, *90*, 1–10. [CrossRef]
49. Mitek, M.; Anyzewska, A.; Wawrzyniak, A. Estimated dietary intakes of nitrates in vegetarians compared to a traditional diet in Poland and acceptable daily intakes: Is there a risk? *Rocz. Panstw. Zakl. Hig.* **2013**, *64*, 105–109.
50. De Filippis, F.; Vannini, L.; La Storia, A.; Laghi, L.; Piombino, P.; Stellato, G.; Serrazanetti, D.I.; Gozzi, G.; Turroni, S.; Ferrocino, I.; et al. The same microbiota and a potentially discriminant metabolome in the saliva of omnivore, ovo-lacto-vegetarian and Vegan individuals. *PLoS ONE* **2014**, *9*, e112373. [CrossRef]
51. Hansen, T.H.; Kern, T.; Bak, E.G.; Kashani, A.; Allin, K.H.; Nielsen, T.; Hansen, T.; Pedersen, O. Impact of a vegan diet on the human salivary microbiota. *Sci. Rep.* **2018**, *8*, 5847. [CrossRef] [PubMed]
52. Tribble, G.D.; Angelov, N.; Weltman, R.; Wang, B.Y.; Eswaran, S.V.; Gay, I.C.; Parthasarathy, K.; Dao, D.V.; Richardson, K.N.; Ismail, N.M.; et al. Frequency of Tongue Cleaning Impacts the Human Tongue Microbiome Composition and Enterosalivary Circulation of Nitrate. *Front. Cell. Infect. Microbiol.* **2019**, *9*, 39. [CrossRef] [PubMed]
53. Quirynen, M.; Dadamio, J.; Van den Velde, S.; De Smit, M.; Dekeyser, C.; Van Tornout, M.; Vandekerckhove, B. Characteristics of 2000 patients who visited a halitosis clinic. *J. Clin. Periodontol.* **2009**, *36*, 970–975. [CrossRef] [PubMed]
54. Graudal, N.A.; Hubeck-Graudal, T.; Jurgens, G. Effects of low sodium diet versus high sodium diet on blood pressure, renin, aldosterone, catecholamines, cholesterol, and triglyceride. *Cochrane Database Syst. Rev.* **2017**, *4*, CD004022. [CrossRef] [PubMed]

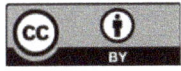

© 2019 by the authors. Licensee MDPI, Basel, Switzerland. This article is an open access article distributed under the terms and conditions of the Creative Commons Attribution (CC BY) license (http://creativecommons.org/licenses/by/4.0/).

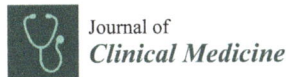

Review

Tools of *Aggregatibacter actinomycetemcomitans* to Evade the Host Response

Jan Oscarsson [1], **Rolf Claesson** [1], **Mark Lindholm** [1], **Carola Höglund Åberg** [2] **and Anders Johansson** [2,*]

1. Department of Odontology, Oral Microbiology, Umeå University, S-90187 Umeå, Sweden
2. Department of Odontology, Molecular Periodontology, Umeå University, S-901 87 Umeå, Sweden
* Correspondence: anders.p.johansson@umu.se

Received: 26 June 2019; Accepted: 18 July 2019; Published: 22 July 2019

Abstract: Periodontitis is an infection-induced inflammatory disease that affects the tooth supporting tissues, i.e., bone and connective tissues. The initiation and progression of this disease depend on dysbiotic ecological changes in the oral microbiome, thereby affecting the severity of disease through multiple immune-inflammatory responses. *Aggregatibacter actinomycetemcomitans* is a facultative anaerobic Gram-negative bacterium associated with such cellular and molecular mechanisms associated with the pathogenesis of periodontitis. In the present review, we outline virulence mechanisms that help the bacterium to escape the host response. These properties include invasiveness, secretion of exotoxins, serum resistance, and release of outer membrane vesicles. Virulence properties of *A. actinomycetemcomitans* that can contribute to treatment resistance in the infected individuals and upon translocation to the circulation, also induce pathogenic mechanisms associated with several systemic diseases.

Keywords: *Aggregatibacter actinomycetemcomitans*; invasiveness; leukotoxin; cytolethal distending toxin; serum resistance; outer membrane vesicles

1. Introduction

Aggregatibacter actinomycetemcomitans is an opportunistic pathogen associated with aggressive forms of periodontitis that affect young individuals [1,2]. The bacterium colonizes the oral mucosa early in life and is inherited by vertical transmission from close relatives [3]. Colonization of *A. actinomycetemcomitans* on the mucosa is not associated with disease but is considered as a risk factor for translocation of the organism to the gingival margin [4]. Bacteria that colonize this ecological niche have the potential to initiate periodontal diseases if they are allowed to stay, proliferate, and express virulence factors [5,6]. *A. actinomycetemcomitans* is a facultative anaerobic Gram-negative bacterium with the capacity to produce a number of virulence factors, and it exhibits a large genetic diversity [2,7]. This bacterium is an early colonizer in the disease process, and resists oxygen and hydrogen peroxide, but is later often replaced by more strict anaerobes in the deep periodontal pocket [1]. In addition to colonizing the oral cavity, systemic translocation of this bacterium is frequently reported [8,9]. *A. actinomycetemcomitans* expresses adhesins that allow colonization of to the tooth surface and the oral epithelium, as well as to mature supragingival plaque [2]. The bacterium is described as an organism that utilizes the other inhabitants in the biofilm for its survival and utilizes metabolic products from other inhabitants of the biofilm for survival and growth [1]. In addition, it is suggested that *A. actinomycetemcomitans* can promote the overgrowth of other bacterial species, which can result in local host dysbiosis and susceptibility to infection [1]. The association of *A. actinomycetemcomitans* to systemic diseases includes endocarditis, cardiovascular diseases, diabetes, Alzheimer´s disease, and rheumatoid arthritis [10–15]. The mechanisms behind these associations are not known, but several virulence properties of *A. actinomycetemcomitans*, such as tissue invasiveness, exotoxin production, serum resistance, and outer membrane vesicle secretion are potential weapons [16–19]. In the sections below, we will further address and discuss the tools behind the ability of this bacterium to evade and suppress the host immune response. The aim of the present review is to identify and describe virulence mechanisms of *A. actinomycetemcomitans*, which are associated with immune subversion, as well as bacterial pathogenicity.

2. Invasive Properties

Invasion of periodontal tissues by different bacterial species has been reported in human periodontitis for several decades [20–22]. The study by Saglie and co-workers [22] observed the prevalence and gingival localization of *A. actinomycetemcomitans* in periodontal lesions of young patients. Transmission electron microscopic examination showed microcolonies of small Gram-negative rods in the connective tissue, as well as single bacterial cells between collagen fibers and in areas of cell debris [20]. In addition to these intra-tissue bacterial cells, bacteria were also found within phagocytic cells, which had invaded the gingival connective tissue. More recent studies have demonstrated invasion of *A. actinomycetemcomitans* into epithelial cells in vitro [23–25]. Interestingly, some *A. actinomycetemcomitans* genotypes have been suggested to have different tissue invasive-properties [23]. If this difference in invasive properties interferes with the ability of *A. actinomycetemcomitans* to cause various periodontal or systemic diseases is not known.

A number of *A. actinomycetemcomitans* factors that likely contribute to host cell invasion have been elucidated. These include the *tad* (tight adherence) gene locus, which mediates adhesion and is required for virulence in a rat model for periodontal disease [26]. OmpA1 (also known as Omp29) is associated with the entry of *A. actinomycetemcomitans* into gingival epithelial cells by up-regulating F-actin rearrangement via the FAK signaling pathway [27], and Omp100 (also known as ApiA) promotes adhesion of *A. actinomycetemcomitans* cells, and their invasion of human gingival keratinocytes [28,29]. It has also been described that bacteria that express a cytolethal distending toxin, such as *A. actinomycetemcomitans*, can cause disruption of the epithelial barrier and promote tissue invasion [30]. A role of *A. actinomycetemcomitans* invasion in immune modulation is supported by in vitro evidence of a subsequent induction of pro-inflammatory cytokine production, and/or apoptosis, in epithelial cells and macrophage-like cells, respectively [31,32].

Severe extra-oral infections caused by *A. actinomycetemcomitans* include brain abscesses, meningitis, septicemia, urinary tract infections, osteomyelitis, and endocarditis [18,33–35]. Whether the systemic translocation through the epithelial barrier is due to an active invasive process, or a result of a passive leakage into the blood stream is not known [36,37]. Bacterial invasion of the periodontal tissues has been suggested as a relevant stage in the etiopathogenesis of periodontal disease, however, there is insufficient evidence to support or exclude this mechanism as a key step in periodontal disease [38,39]. Despite the lack of conclusive studies, the invasive properties of *A. actinomycetemcomitans* have the potential to help the bacterium to evade mechanical and chemical strategies immune responses, and mechanical or chemical eradication strategies [40] (Figure 1). If these properties of the bacterium contribute to systemic translocation and survival has not yet been studied. Evidently, major reasons for bacteremia caused by oral bacteria such as *A. actinomycetemcomitans* are gingival inflammation and mechanical manipulation [41].

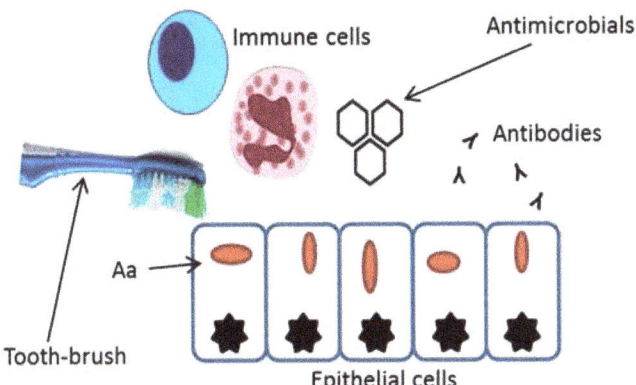

Figure 1. Invasion of *A. actinomycetemcomitans* into epithelial cells can protect the bacterial cells from mechanical removal, antibiotics, immune cell phagocytosis, and antibody binding.

3. Production of Exotoxins

A. actinomycetemcomitans is the only bacterium colonizing the oral cavity known to produce two exotoxins [42,43], leukotoxin (LtxA) that specifically induces killing of human leukocytes, and a cytolethal distending toxin (CDT), which is a genotoxin, causing growth arrest by affecting DNA in proliferating cells [16,44]. Both toxins are highly conserved and occur also in several other Gram-negative pathogens [45,46]. As a sign of the large genetic diversity of *A. actinomycetemcomitans*, there are strains, representing various genotypes, which produce highly different levels of these toxins [2,6,47]. All hitherto studied *A. actinomycetemcomitans* strains carry a complete *ltxCABD* gene locus, encoding for LtxA, activation and secretion [6]. Mutations, i.e., deletions and insertions in the *ltx* promoter region have been shown to influence leukotoxin production in *A. actinomycetemcomitans* [48–50]. The so called JP2 genotype, which harbors a 530-bp deletion in the *ltx* promoter region is well studied, and known to be strongly associated with disease risk in the individuals carrying it [5,6,51]. Its high LtxA production is considered to be an important factor for the enhanced pathogenicity of this genotype [52].

LtxA induces several pathogenic mechanisms in human leukocytes that can all be linked to the progression of periodontal disease [16]. A substantial humoral immune response against LtxA is initiated in all the infected individuals [53,54]. LtxA kills immune cells and protects the bacterium from phagocytic killing [55]. Neutrophils exposed to LtxA activate degranulation, concomitant with an extracellular release of proteolytic enzymes and metalloproteases, such as elastase and metallproteases [56,57]. LtxA can also affect human macrophages by activating the inflammasome complex, which results in the activation and secretion of pro-inflammatory enzymes (i.e., IL-1β and IL-18) [58]. In this context, an interesting observation was recently made that *A. actinomycetemcomitans* expresses an outer membrane lipoprotein, which binds host cytokines, including IL-1β [59]. The IL-1β binding protein was designated bacterial interleukin receptor I (BilRI) and has the ability to internalize IL-1β into the viable bacterial biofilm [60]. Taken together, the abilities of LtxA to cause a proteolytic environment that can degrade immunoproteins, internalize inflammatory proteins, and kill immune cells may all contribute to the survival of *A. actinomycetemcomitans* in the infected host.

The CDT is expressed by a majority of *A. actinomycetemcomitans* genotypes, even though some of them lack a complete gene operon for expression of an active holo-toxin [45]. In vitro and in vivo studies have shown that CDT affects cellular physiology involved in inflammation, immune response modulation, and causes tissue damage [61,62]. The holo-toxin consists of three subunits (CdtA, B, and C) and is transported to the nucleus of the mammalian target cells [63]. Cells exposed for CDT induce a growth arrest followed by apoptotic cell death [44,63]. In cultures of periodontal fibroblasts, CDT induces expression of cytokines and the osteoclast activating protein, receptor activator of nuclear factor kappa-B ligand (RANKL) [64,65]. The role of CDT in the pathogenesis of periodontitis is not entirely clear, and the literature contains studies that demonstrate an association, as well as those reporting no correlation [42,66,67].

Together LtxA and CDT can act as strong weapons against the immune response raised against *A. actinomycetemcomitans*. They can cause an imbalance in the host response by activating inflammation, killing immune cells, affecting antigen presenting cells, and inhibiting lymphocyte proliferation (Figure 2). The impact of these exotoxins in the pathogenesis of periodontal disease is apparent, whereas their role in systemic diseases is not known. However, LtxA-exposed neutrophils do release net-like structures and express patterns of citrullinated proteins that are similar to those observed in synovial fluid from inflamed joints [12,68]. Moreover, antibiotic treatment of a periodontitis patient, infected with the highly leukotoxic JP2 genotype of *A. actinomycetemcomitans*, and suffering from rheumatoid arthritis, was also cured of the joint pain after the treatment [69]. These observations indicate that *A. actinomycetemcomitans* is an interesting organism in the etiopathogenesis of rheumatoid arthritis.

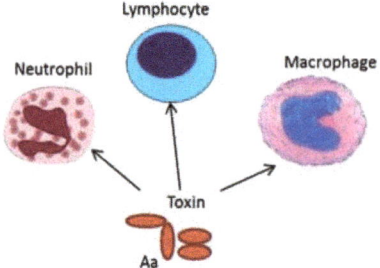

Figure 2. Expression of exotoxins can result in resistance of *A. actinomycetemcomitans* to phagocytosis and neutrophil degranulation. The cytolethal distending toxin (CDT) can cause inhibited proliferation of stimulated lymphocytes, and LtxA induces an inflammatory cell death in the antigen presenting cells, macrophages, and monocytes.

4. Serum Resistance

Serum resistance represents an important virulence factor of bacteria that enter into the bloodstream and cause infection, allowing the bacterial cells to evade the innate immune defense mechanisms present in serum, including the complement system and antimicrobial peptides [70–72]. The recognition of bacterial products mediating serum resistance, therefore, represents an approach to the vaccine and drug development [73,74]. Resistance to complement-mediated killing by human serum appears to be important for *A. actinomycetemcomitans* virulence, and is a common characteristic among strains of this species, although they typically do not form capsules [28,75]. The outer membrane protein, Omp100 (ApiA), was earlier demonstrated to be important for serum resistance in some serotype b and d strains and to physically interact with and trap the alternative complement pathway negative regulator, Factor H, in vitro [28,76] (Figure 3).

Evidently, Omps produced by *A. actinomycetemcomitans* strains are immuno-reactive in the human host [77]. As the presence of antibodies towards bacterial antigens such as Omps is a known trigger of classical complement activation [78], serum resistance of *A. actinomycetemcomitans* strains would be expected to also include mechanisms interacting with this activation. We recently presented evidence that the major outer membrane protein, OmpA1, is critical for serum survival in the *A. actinomycetemcomitans* serotype a model strain, D7SS [17]. Outer membrane integrity may be one mechanism behind OmpA-mediated serum resistance in Gram-negative bacteria [79]. Interestingly, serum resistant *ompA1* mutants were fortuitously obtained, which expressed increased levels of the paralogue, OmpA2. Thus, OmpA2 can apparently operate as a functional homologue to OmpA1 in *A. actinomycetemcomitans*, and both proteins seemingly act, at least partly by binding and trapping of C4-binding protein [17] (Figure 3), which is an inhibitor of classical and mannose-binding lectin (MBL) complement activation [80]. Further to these activation pathways, alternative complement activation is needed to fully eliminate serum-sensitive *ompA* mutant *A. actinomycetemcomitans* derivatives [17]. It is plausible that serum resistance in this species, similar to in *Acinetobacter baumanii* [81], is highly complex and relies on a large number of gene products, including host factors. For example, whether cleavage of the complement molecule C3 by elastase [82], which release is triggered by leukotoxin [57], may contribute to *A. actinomycetemcomitans* serum resistance is not known. Moreover, albeit *A. actinomycetemcomitans* strains are ubiquitously serum resistant, strains not expressing their immunodominant, serotype-specific polysaccharide (S-PA) antigen are occasionally isolated [83]. As speculated previously [83], the lack of S-PA expression may represent a mechanism to evade from antibody-based host responses, which could be advantageous in blood circulation. However, an inconsistency with this notion is that the absence of S-PA expression in *A. actinomycetemcomitans* appears to be scarce.

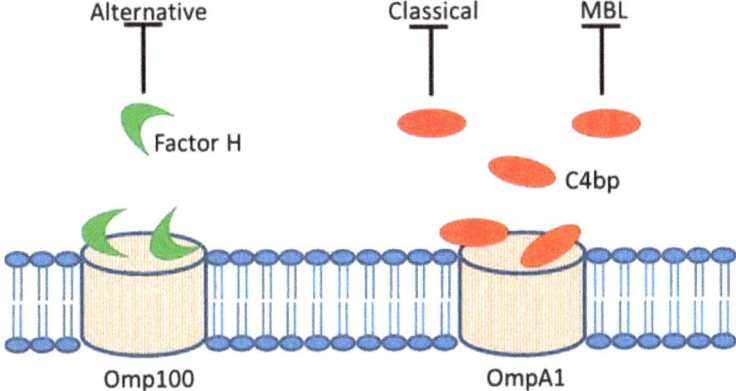

Figure 3. Serum resistance. In vitro evidence supports that *A. actinomycetemcomitans* outer membrane proteins, Omp100 and OmpA1, may allow trapping of soluble repressors of complement activation, i.e., Factor H and C4 binding protein (C4bp), respectively. This would result in downregulation of the alternative, classical, and mannose-binding lectin (MBL) pathway of complement activation.

5. Outer Membrane Vesicles

Outer Membrane Vesicles (OMVs) of Gram-negative bacteria are spherical membrane-enclosed nanostructures that are released from the outer membrane. They can operate as a fundamental mechanism for discharging proteins and additional bacterial components into the surrounding environment and to target host cells [84,85]. Evidence from in vitro experiments shows that *A. actinomycetemcomitans* OMVs can deliver an abundance of biologically active virulence factors to host cells, and which can modulate the immune response (Figure 4).

One such example is CDT, which is delivered into HeLa cells and human gingival fibroblasts via OMVs [86]. OMVs are also involved in the export of LtxA, peptidoglycan-associated lipoprotein (Pal), and the chaperonin GroEL to host cells [87–90]. Proteomics and Western blot analysis of *A. actinomycetemcomitans* OMVs has identified additional proteins that can contribute to evasion of the immune defense, including the IL1β-binding lipoprotein, BilRI, the outer membrane proteins Omp100, OmpA1, and OmpA2, and a Factor H-binding protein homologue [17,91,92]. A functional role in the interaction with complement by vesicles is supported by observations that *A. actinomycetemcomitans* OMVs in an OmpA1-dependent manner can bind to the classical and MBL complement inhibitor, C4-binding protein [17]. It has also been demonstrated that *A. actinomycetemcomitans* OMVs can carry small molecules, including lipopolysaccharide (LPS), which can interact with complement [93]. LPS may also play a role in the observed binding of *A. actinomycetemcomitans* OMVs to IL-8 [94]. Evidence that *A. actinomycetemcomitans* OMVs carry NOD1- and NOD2-active peptidoglycan, which can be internalized into non-phagocytic human cells including gingival fibroblasts [19], reveals a role of the vesicles as a trigger of innate immunity. Moreover, OMV-dependent release of microRNA-size small RNAs (msRNAs), may potentially represent a mechanism to transfer a novel class of bacterial signaling molecules into host cells [95]. It is not completely understood how *A. actinomycetemcomitans* OMVs may physically interact with and/or enter into human host cells to enhance bacterial evasion of the immune defense. The OMVs appear to enter into human cells via clathrin-mediated endocytosis [19,96], but can also fuse with host membranes in a process dependent on cholesterol [86]. Toxins exported via OMVs can function as adhesins in receptor-mediated endocytosis of the vesicles [97], albeit neither CDT nor leukotoxin are required *per se* for the OMV uptake into host cells [86,87]. Concomitantly, although LtxA has an apparent localization on the *A. actinomycetemcomitans* OMV surface, its receptor LFA-1 is not required for delivering the toxin into host cells [98].

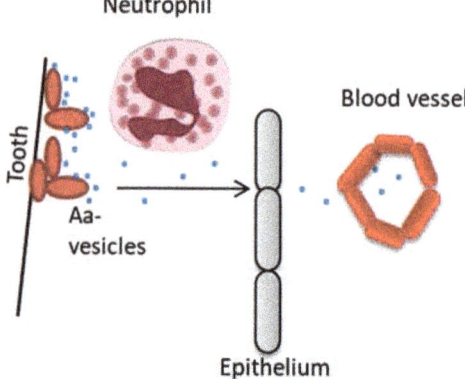

Figure 4. Release of outer membrane vesicles may serve as protection of *A. actinomycetemcomitans* from phagocytic- and serum killing, and also as a means to transport virulence factors to tissues that not are in close contact with the infecting bacteria.

6. Conclusions

We have summarized current knowledge regarding major attributes and strategies of *A. actinomycetemcomitans*, allowing this organism to evade the host response. Without doubt, the numerous virulence properties of *A. actinomycetemcomitans* can be linked to the pathogenesis of periodontal disease [99]. Utilization of these properties for systemic translocation of *A. actinomycetemcomitans* and its subsequent survival in this new environment has been excellently summarized and illustrated [1,100]. It is today hypothesized that the virulence characteristics of *A. actinomycetemcomitans* allow this organism to induce an immune subversion that tip the balance from homeostasis over to disease in oral and/or extra-oral sites [101]. Hence, in order to prohibit the negative systemic consequences that are associated with periodontitis, successful treatment in an early phase of the disease is fundamental. Development of specific diagnostic tools for assessment of periodontal pathogens and inflammatory components in the saliva of young individuals might make it possible to prevent the disease before its onset.

Author Contributions: Conceptualization, A.J., J.O. and R.C.; writing—original draft preparation, A.J. and J.O.; writing—review and editing, A.J., J.O., R.C., M.L., and C.H.Å.; funding acquisition, A.J., M.L. and J.O.; supervision, C.H.Å., R.C., A.J. and, J.O.

Funding: This work was supported by TUA grants from the County Council of Västerbotten, Sweden (to J.O. and A.J.), by funds from Insamlingsstiftelsen, Medical Faculty, Umeå University (to J.O. and A.J.), and from Svenska Tandläkare-sällskapet, Kempe Foundation, and Thuréus Foundation (to M.L.).

Conflicts of Interest: The authors declare no conflicts of interest.

References

1. Fine, D.H.; Patil, A.G.; Velusamy, S.K. *Aggregatibacter actinomycetemcomitans* (*Aa*) Under the Radar: Myths and Misunderstandings of *Aa* and Its Role in Aggressive Periodontitis. *Front. Immunol.* **2019**, *10*, 728. [CrossRef] [PubMed]
2. Henderson, B.; Ward, J.M.; Ready, D. *Aggregatibacter* (*Actinobacillus*) *actinomycetemcomitans*: A triple A* periodontopathogen? *Periodontol. 2000* **2010**, *54*, 78–105. [CrossRef] [PubMed]
3. Könönen, E.; Muller, H.P. Microbiology of aggressive periodontitis. *Periodontol. 2000* **2014**, *65*, 46–78. [CrossRef] [PubMed]
4. Höglund Åberg, C.; Kelk, P.; Johansson, A. *Aggregatibacter actinomycetemcomitans*: Virulence of its leukotoxin and association with aggressive periodontitis. *Virulence* **2015**, *6*, 188–195. [CrossRef] [PubMed]
5. Haubek, D.; Ennibi, O.K.; Poulsen, K.; Vaeth, M.; Poulsen, S.; Kilian, M. Risk of aggressive periodontitis in adolescent carriers of the JP2 clone of *Aggregatibacter* (*Actinobacillus*) *actinomycetemcomitans* in Morocco: A prospective longitudinal cohort study. *Lancet* **2008**, *371*, 237–242. [CrossRef]
6. Höglund Åberg, C.; Kwamin, F.; Claesson, R.; Dahlen, G.; Johansson, A.; Haubek, D. Progression of attachment loss is strongly associated with presence of the JP2 genotype of *Aggregatibacter actinomycetemcomitans*: A prospective cohort study of a young adolescent population. *J. Clin. Periodontol.* **2014**, *41*, 232–241. [CrossRef] [PubMed]
7. Kittichotirat, W.; Bumgarner, R.E.; Chen, C. Evolutionary Divergence of *Aggregatibacter actinomycetemcomitans*. *J. Dent. Res.* **2016**, *95*, 94–101. [CrossRef]
8. Paju, S.; Carlson, P.; Jousimies-Somer, H.; Asikainen, S. *Actinobacillus actinomycetemcomitans* and *Haemophilus aphrophilus* in systemic and nonoral infections in Finland. *APMIS* **2003**, *111*, 653–657. [CrossRef]
9. van Winkelhoff, A.J.; Slots, J. *Actinobacillus actinomycetemcomitans* and *Porphyromonas gingivalis* in nonoral infections. *Periodontol. 2000* **1999**, *20*, 122–135. [CrossRef]
10. Demmer, R.T.; Jacobs, D.R., Jr.; Singh, R.; Zuk, A.; Rosenbaum, M.; Papapanou, P.N.; Desvarieux, M. Periodontal Bacteria and Prediabetes Prevalence in ORIGINS: The Oral Infections, Glucose Intolerance, and Insulin Resistance Study. *J. Dent. Res.* **2015**, *94*, 201S–211S. [CrossRef]
11. Diaz-Zuniga, J.; Munoz, Y.; Melgar-Rodriguez, S.; More, J.; Bruna, B.; Lobos, P.; Monasterio, G.; Vernal, R.; Paula-Lima, A. Serotype b of *Aggregatibacter actinomycetemcomitans* triggers pro-inflammatory responses and amyloid beta secretion in hippocampal cells: A novel link between periodontitis and Alzheimer's disease? *J. Oral Microbiol.* **2019**, *11*, 1586423. [CrossRef] [PubMed]
12. Konig, M.F.; Abusleme, L.; Reinholdt, J.; Palmer, R.J.; Teles, R.P.; Sampson, K.; Rosen, A.; Nigrovic, P.A.; Sokolove, J.; Giles, J.T.; et al. *Aggregatibacter actinomycetemcomitans*-induced hypercitrullination links periodontal infection to autoimmunity in rheumatoid arthritis. *Sci. Transl. Med.* **2016**, *8*, 369ra176. [CrossRef] [PubMed]
13. Laugisch, O.; Johnen, A.; Maldonado, A.; Ehmke, B.; Burgin, W.; Olsen, I.; Potempa, J.; Sculean, A.; Duning, T.; Eick, S. Periodontal Pathogens and Associated Intrathecal Antibodies in Early Stages of Alzheimer's Disease. *J. Alzheimers Dis.* **2018**, *66*, 105–114. [CrossRef] [PubMed]
14. Liljestrand, J.M.; Paju, S.; Pietiainen, M.; Buhlin, K.; Persson, G.R.; Nieminen, M.S.; Sinisalo, J.; Mantyla, P.; Pussinen, P.J. Immunologic burden links periodontitis to acute coronary syndrome. *Atherosclerosis* **2018**, *268*, 177–184. [CrossRef] [PubMed]
15. Revest, M.; Egmann, G.; Cattoir, V.; Tattevin, P. HACEK endocarditis: State-of-the-art. *Expert Rev. Anti-Infect. Ther.* **2016**, *14*, 523–530. [CrossRef] [PubMed]
16. Johansson, A. *Aggregatibacter actinomycetemcomitans* leukotoxin: A powerful tool with capacity to cause imbalance in the host inflammatory response. *Toxins* **2011**, *3*, 242–259. [CrossRef] [PubMed]
17. Lindholm, M.; Min Aung, K.; Nyunt Wai, S.; Oscarsson, J. Role of OmpA1 and OmpA2 in *Aggregatibacter actinomycetemcomitans* and *Aggregatibacter aphrophilus* serum resistance. *J. Oral Microbiol.* **2019**, *11*, 1536192. [CrossRef] [PubMed]
18. Raja, M.; Ummer, F.; Dhivakar, C.P. *Aggregatibacter actinomycetemcomitans*—A tooth killer? *J. Clin. Diagn. Res.* **2014**, *8*, ZE13–ZE16. [CrossRef]
19. Thay, B.; Damm, A.; Kufer, T.A.; Wai, S.N.; Oscarsson, J. *Aggregatibacter actinomycetemcomitans* outer membrane vesicles are internalized in human host cells and trigger NOD1- and NOD2-dependent NF-kappaB activation. *Infect. Immun.* **2014**, *82*, 4034–4046. [CrossRef]

20. Christersson, L.A.; Albini, B.; Zambon, J.J.; Wikesjo, U.M.; Genco, R.J. Tissue localization of *Actinobacillus actinomycetemcomitans* in human periodontitis. I. Light, immunofluorescence and electron microscopic studies. *J. Periodontol.* **1987**, *58*, 529–539. [CrossRef]
21. Christersson, L.A.; Wikesjo, U.M.; Albini, B.; Zambon, J.J.; Genco, R.J. Tissue localization of *Actinobacillus actinomycetemcomitans* in human periodontitis. II. Correlation between immunofluorescence and culture techniques. *J. Periodontol.* **1987**, *58*, 540–545. [CrossRef] [PubMed]
22. Saglie, F.R.; Marfany, A.; Camargo, P. Intragingival occurrence of *Actinobacillus actinomycetemcomitans* and *Bacteroides gingivalis* in active destructive periodontal lesions. *J. Periodontol.* **1988**, *59*, 259–265. [CrossRef] [PubMed]
23. Lepine, G.; Caudry, S.; DiRienzo, J.M.; Ellen, R.P. Epithelial cell invasion by *Actinobacillus actinomycetemcomitans* strains from restriction fragment-length polymorphism groups associated with juvenile periodontitis or carrier status. *Oral Microbiol. Immunol.* **1998**, *13*, 341–347. [CrossRef] [PubMed]
24. Meyer, D.H.; Sreenivasan, P.K.; Fives-Taylor, P.M. Evidence for invasion of a human oral cell line by *Actinobacillus actinomycetemcomitans*. *Infect. Immun.* **1991**, *59*, 2719–2726. [PubMed]
25. Meyer, D.H.; Lippmann, J.E.; Fives-Taylor, P.M. Invasion of epithelial cells by *Actinobacillus actinomycetemcomitans*: A dynamic, multistep process. *Infect. Immun.* **1996**, *64*, 2988–2997.
26. Schreiner, H.C.; Sinatra, K.; Kaplan, J.B.; Furgang, D.; Kachlany, S.C.; Planet, P.J.; Perez, B.A.; Figurski, D.H.; Fine, D.H. Tight-adherence genes of *Actinobacillus actinomycetemcomitans* are required for virulence in a rat model. *Proc. Natl. Acad. Sci. USA* **2003**, *100*, 7295–7300. [CrossRef] [PubMed]
27. Kajiya, M.; Komatsuzawa, H.; Papantonakis, A.; Seki, M.; Makihira, S.; Ouhara, K.; Kusumoto, Y.; Murakami, S.; Taubman, M.A.; Kawai, T. *Aggregatibacter actinomycetemcomitans* Omp29 is associated with bacterial entry to gingival epithelial cells by F-actin rearrangement. *PLoS ONE* **2011**, *6*, e18287. [CrossRef]
28. Asakawa, R.; Komatsuzawa, H.; Kawai, T.; Yamada, S.; Goncalves, R.B.; Izumi, S.; Fujiwara, T.; Nakano, Y.; Suzuki, N.; Uchida, Y.; et al. Outer membrane protein 100, a versatile virulence factor of *Actinobacillus actinomycetemcomitans*. *Mol. Microbiol.* **2003**, *50*, 1125–1139. [CrossRef]
29. Yue, G.; Kaplan, J.B.; Furgang, D.; Mansfield, K.G.; Fine, D.H. A second *Aggregatibacter actinomycetemcomitans* autotransporter adhesin exhibits specificity for buccal epithelial cells in humans and Old World primates. *Infect. Immun.* **2007**, *75*, 4440–4448. [CrossRef]
30. DiRienzo, J.M. Breaking the Gingival Epithelial Barrier: Role of the *Aggregatibacter actinomycetemcomitans* Cytolethal Distending Toxin in Oral Infectious Disease. *Cells* **2014**, *3*, 476–499. [CrossRef]
31. Dickinson, B.C.; Moffatt, C.E.; Hagerty, D.; Whitmore, S.E.; Brown, T.A.; Graves, D.T.; Lamont, R.J. Interaction of oral bacteria with gingival epithelial cell multilayers. *Mol. Oral Microbiol.* **2011**, *26*, 210–220. [CrossRef] [PubMed]
32. Okinaga, T.; Ariyoshi, W.; Nishihara, T. *Aggregatibacter actinomycetemcomitans* Invasion Induces Interleukin-1beta Production Through Reactive Oxygen Species and Cathepsin B. *J. Interferon. Cytokine Res.* **2015**, *35*, 431–440. [CrossRef] [PubMed]
33. Rahamat-Langendoen, J.C.; van Vonderen, M.G.; Engstrom, L.J.; Manson, W.L.; van Winkelhoff, A.J.; Mooi-Kokenberg, E.A. Brain abscess associated with *Aggregatibacter actinomycetemcomitans*: Case report and review of literature. *J. Clin. Periodontol.* **2011**, *38*, 702–706. [CrossRef] [PubMed]
34. Stepanovic, S.; Tosic, T.; Savic, B.; Jovanovic, M.; K'Ouas, G.; Carlier, J.P. Brain abscess due to *Actinobacillus actinomycetemcomitans*. *APMIS* **2005**, *113*, 225–228. [CrossRef] [PubMed]
35. Tang, G.; Kitten, T.; Munro, C.L.; Wellman, G.C.; Mintz, K.P. EmaA, a potential virulence determinant of *Aggregatibacter actinomycetemcomitans* in infective endocarditis. *Infect. Immun.* **2008**, *76*, 2316–2324. [CrossRef]
36. Doran, K.S.; Banerjee, A.; Disson, O.; Lecuit, M. Concepts and mechanisms: Crossing host barriers. *Cold Spring Harb. Perspect. Med.* **2013**, *3*. [CrossRef] [PubMed]
37. Ribet, D.; Cossart, P. How bacterial pathogens colonize their hosts and invade deeper tissues. *Microbes Infect.* **2015**, *17*, 173–183. [CrossRef]
38. Ji, S.; Choi, Y.S.; Choi, Y. Bacterial invasion and persistence: Critical events in the pathogenesis of periodontitis? *J. Periodontal Res.* **2015**, *50*, 570–585. [CrossRef]

39. Mendes, L.; Azevedo, N.F.; Felino, A.; Pinto, M.G. Relationship between invasion of the periodontium by periodontal pathogens and periodontal disease: A systematic review. *Virulence* **2015**, *6*, 208–215. [CrossRef]
40. Eick, S.; Pfister, W. Efficacy of antibiotics against periodontopathogenic bacteria within epithelial cells: An in vitro study. *J. Periodontol.* **2004**, *75*, 1327–1334. [CrossRef]
41. Hirschfeld, J.; Kawai, T. Oral inflammation and bacteremia: Implications for chronic and acute systemic diseases involving major organs. *Cardiovasc. Hematol. Disord. Drug Targets* **2015**, *15*, 70–84. [CrossRef] [PubMed]
42. Höglund Åberg, C.; Antonoglou, G.; Haubek, D.; Kwamin, F.; Claesson, R.; Johansson, A. Cytolethal distending toxin in isolates of *Aggregatibacter actinomycetemcomitans* from Ghanaian adolescents and association with serotype and disease progression. *PLoS ONE* **2013**, *8*, e65781. [CrossRef]
43. Höglund Åberg, C.; Haubek, D.; Kwamin, F.; Johansson, A.; Claesson, R. Leukotoxic activity of *Aggregatibacter actinomycetemcomitans* and periodontal attachment loss. *PLoS ONE* **2014**, *9*, e104095. [CrossRef] [PubMed]
44. Belibasakis, G.N.; Mattsson, A.; Wang, Y.; Chen, C.; Johansson, A. Cell cycle arrest of human gingival fibroblasts and periodontal ligament cells by *Actinobacillus actinomycetemcomitans*: Involvement of the cytolethal distending toxin. *APMIS* **2004**, *112*, 674–685. [CrossRef] [PubMed]
45. Fais, T.; Delmas, J.; Serres, A.; Bonnet, R.; Dalmasso, G. Impact of CDT Toxin on Human Diseases. *Toxins* **2016**, *8*, 220. [CrossRef] [PubMed]
46. Linhartova, I.; Bumba, L.; Masin, J.; Basler, M.; Osicka, R.; Kamanova, J.; Prochazkova, K.; Adkins, I.; Hejnova-Holubova, J.; Sadilkova, L.; et al. RTX proteins: A highly diverse family secreted by a common mechanism. *FEMS Microbiol. Rev.* **2010**, *34*, 1076–1112. [CrossRef] [PubMed]
47. Johansson, A.; Claesson, R.; Hoglund Aberg, C.; Haubek, D.; Oscarsson, J. The cagE gene sequence as a diagnostic marker to identify JP2 and non-JP2 highly leukotoxic *Aggregatibacter actinomycetemcomitans* serotype b strains. *J. Periodontal. Res.* **2017**, *52*, 903–912. [CrossRef]
48. Brogan, J.M.; Lally, E.T.; Poulsen, K.; Kilian, M.; Demuth, D.R. Regulation of *Actinobacillus actinomycetemcomitans* leukotoxin expression: Analysis of the promoter regions of leukotoxic and minimally leukotoxic strains. *Infect. Immun.* **1994**, *62*, 501–508.
49. Claesson, R.; Gudmundson, J.; Höglund Åberg, C.; Haubek, D.; Johansson, A. Detection of a 640-bp deletion in the *Aggregatibacter actinomycetemcomitans* leukotoxin promoter region in isolates from an adolescent of Ethiopian origin. *J. Oral Microbiol.* **2015**, *7*, 26974. [CrossRef]
50. He, T.; Hayashi, J.; Yamamoto, M.; Ishikawa, I. Genotypic characterization of *Actinobacillus actinomycetemcomitans* isolated from periodontitis patients by arbitrarily primed polymerase chain reaction. *J. Periodontol.* **1998**, *69*, 69–75. [CrossRef]
51. Ennibi, O.K.; Claesson, R.; Akkaoui, S.; Reddahi, S.; Kwamin, F.; Haubek, D.; Johansson, A. High salivary levels of JP2 genotype of *Aggregatibacter actinomycetemcomitans* is associated with clinical attachment loss in Moroccan adolescents. *Clin. Exp. Dent. Res.* **2019**, *5*, 44–51. [CrossRef] [PubMed]
52. Haubek, D.; Johansson, A. Pathogenicity of the highly leukotoxic JP2 clone of *Aggregatibacter actinomycetemcomitans* and its geographic dissemination and role in aggressive periodontitis. *J. Oral Microbiol.* **2014**, *6*. [CrossRef]
53. Brage, M.; Holmlund, A.; Johansson, A. Humoral immune response to *Aggregatibacter actinomycetemcomitans* leukotoxin. *J. Periodontal. Res.* **2011**, *46*, 170–175. [CrossRef] [PubMed]
54. Johansson, A.; Buhlin, K.; Sorsa, T.; Pussinen, P.J. Systemic *Aggregatibacter actinomycetemcomitans* Leukotoxin-Neutralizing Antibodies in Periodontitis. *J. Periodontol.* **2017**, *88*, 122–129. [CrossRef] [PubMed]
55. Johansson, A.; Sandstrom, G.; Claesson, R.; Hanstrom, L.; Kalfas, S. Anaerobic neutrophil-dependent killing of *Actinobacillus actinomycetemcomitans* in relation to the bacterial leukotoxicity. *Eur. J. Oral Sci.* **2000**, *108*, 136–146. [CrossRef] [PubMed]
56. Claesson, R.; Johansson, A.; Belibasakis, G.; Hanstrom, L.; Kalfas, S. Release and activation of matrix metalloproteinase 8 from human neutrophils triggered by the leukotoxin of *Actinobacillus actinomycetemcomitans*. *J. Periodontal. Res.* **2002**, *37*, 353–359. [CrossRef] [PubMed]
57. Johansson, A.; Claesson, R.; Hänström, L.; Sandström, G.; Kalfas, S. Polymorphonuclear leukocyte degranulation induced by leukotoxin from *Actinobacillus actinomycetemcomitans*. *J. Periodontal. Res.* **2000**, *35*, 85–92. [CrossRef] [PubMed]

58. Kelk, P.; Abd, H.; Claesson, R.; Sandström, G.; Sjöstedt, A.; Johansson, A. Cellular and molecular response of human macrophages exposed to *Aggregatibacter actinomycetemcomitans* leukotoxin. *Cell Death Dis.* **2011**, *2*, e126. [CrossRef]
59. Ahlstrand, T.; Tuominen, H.; Beklen, A.; Torittu, A.; Oscarsson, J.; Sormunen, R.; Pollanen, M.T.; Permi, P.; Ihalin, R. A novel intrinsically disordered outer membrane lipoprotein of *Aggregatibacter actinomycetemcomitans* binds various cytokines and plays a role in biofilm response to interleukin-1beta and interleukin-8. *Virulence* **2017**, *8*, 115–134. [CrossRef]
60. Paino, A.; Ahlstrand, T.; Nuutila, J.; Navickaite, I.; Lahti, M.; Tuominen, H.; Valimaa, H.; Lamminmaki, U.; Pollanen, M.T.; Ihalin, R. Identification of a novel bacterial outer membrane interleukin-1Beta-binding protein from *Aggregatibacter actinomycetemcomitans*. *PLoS ONE* **2013**, *8*, e70509. [CrossRef]
61. Belibasakis, G.N.; Bostanci, N. Inflammatory and bone remodeling responses to the cytolethal distending toxins. *Cells* **2014**, *3*, 236–246. [CrossRef] [PubMed]
62. Kawamoto, D.; Ando-Suguimoto, E.S.; Bueno-Silva, B.; DiRienzo, J.M.; Mayer, M.P. Alteration of Homeostasis in Pre-osteoclasts Induced by *Aggregatibacter actinomycetemcomitans* CDT. *Front. Cell. Infect. Microbiol.* **2016**, *6*, 33. [CrossRef] [PubMed]
63. DiRienzo, J.M. Uptake and processing of the cytolethal distending toxin by mammalian cells. *Toxins* **2014**, *6*, 3098–3116. [CrossRef] [PubMed]
64. Belibasakis, G.N.; Johansson, A.; Wang, Y.; Chen, C.; Kalfas, S.; Lerner, U.H. The cytolethal distending toxin induces receptor activator of NF-kappaB ligand expression in human gingival fibroblasts and periodontal ligament cells. *Infect. Immun.* **2005**, *73*, 342–351. [CrossRef] [PubMed]
65. Belibasakis, G.N.; Johansson, A.; Wang, Y.; Chen, C.; Lagergard, T.; Kalfas, S.; Lerner, U.H. Cytokine responses of human gingival fibroblasts to *Actinobacillus actinomycetemcomitans* cytolethal distending toxin. *Cytokine* **2005**, *30*, 56–63. [CrossRef] [PubMed]
66. Ando, E.S.; De-Gennaro, L.A.; Faveri, M.; Feres, M.; DiRienzo, J.M.; Mayer, M.P. Immune response to cytolethal distending toxin of *Aggregatibacter actinomycetemcomitans* in periodontitis patients. *J. Periodontal. Res.* **2010**, *45*, 471–480. [PubMed]
67. Tan, K.S.; Song, K.P.; Ong, G. Cytolethal distending toxin of *Actinobacillus actinomycetemcomitans*. Occurrence and association with periodontal disease. *J. Periodontal. Res.* **2002**, *37*, 268–272. [CrossRef] [PubMed]
68. Hirschfeld, J.; Roberts, H.M.; Chapple, I.L.; Parcina, M.; Jepsen, S.; Johansson, A.; Claesson, R. Effects of *Aggregatibacter actinomycetemcomitans* leukotoxin on neutrophil migration and extracellular trap formation. *J. Oral Microbiol.* **2016**, *8*, 33070. [CrossRef] [PubMed]
69. Mukherjee, A.; Jantsch, V.; Khan, R.; Hartung, W.; Fischer, R.; Jantsch, J.; Ehrenstein, B.; Konig, M.F.; Andrade, F. Rheumatoid Arthritis-Associated Autoimmunity Due to *Aggregatibacter actinomycetemcomitans* and Its Resolution With Antibiotic Therapy. *Front. Immunol.* **2018**, *9*, 2352. [CrossRef] [PubMed]
70. Abreu, A.G.; Barbosa, A.S. How Escherichia coli Circumvent Complement-Mediated Killing. *Front. Immunol.* **2017**, *8*, 452. [CrossRef] [PubMed]
71. Berends, E.T.; Kuipers, A.; Ravesloot, M.M.; Urbanus, R.T.; Rooijakkers, S.H. Bacteria under stress by complement and coagulation. *FEMS Microbiol. Rev.* **2014**, *38*, 1146–1171. [CrossRef] [PubMed]
72. Hovingh, E.S.; van den Broek, B.; Jongerius, I. Hijacking Complement Regulatory Proteins for Bacterial Immune Evasion. *Front. Microbiol.* **2016**, *7*, 2004. [CrossRef] [PubMed]
73. Jongerius, I.; Schuijt, T.J.; Mooi, F.R.; Pinelli, E. Complement evasion by Bordetella pertussis: Implications for improving current vaccines. *J. Mol. Med.* **2015**, *93*, 395–402. [CrossRef] [PubMed]
74. Vila-Farres, X.; Parra-Millan, R.; Sanchez-Encinales, V.; Varese, M.; Ayerbe-Algaba, R.; Bayo, N.; Guardiola, S.; Pachon-Ibanez, M.E.; Kotev, M.; Garcia, J.; et al. Combating virulence of Gram-negative bacilli by OmpA inhibition. *Sci. Rep.* **2017**, *7*, 14683. [CrossRef] [PubMed]
75. Sundqvist, G.; Johansson, E. Bactericidal effect of pooled human serum on *Bacteroides melaninogenicus*, *Bacteroides asaccharolyticus* and *Actinobacillus actinomycetemcomitans*. *Scand. J. Dent. Res.* **1982**, *90*, 29–36. [CrossRef] [PubMed]
76. Ramsey, M.M.; Whiteley, M. Polymicrobial interactions stimulate resistance to host innate immunity through metabolite perception. *Proc. Natl. Acad. Sci. USA* **2009**, *106*, 1578–1583. [CrossRef] [PubMed]
77. Komatsuzawa, H.; Asakawa, R.; Kawai, T.; Ochiai, K.; Fujiwara, T.; Taubman, M.A.; Ohara, M.; Kurihara, H.; Sugai, M. Identification of six major outer membrane proteins from *Actinobacillus actinomycetemcomitans*. *Gene* **2002**, *288*, 195–201. [CrossRef]

78. Aung, K.M.; Sjostrom, A.E.; von Pawel-Rammingen, U.; Riesbeck, K.; Uhlin, B.E.; Wai, S.N. Naturally Occurring IgG Antibodies Provide Innate Protection against Vibrio cholerae Bacteremia by Recognition of the Outer Membrane Protein U. *J. Innate. Immun.* **2016**, *8*, 269–283. [CrossRef] [PubMed]
79. Confer, A.W.; Ayalew, S. The OmpA family of proteins: Roles in bacterial pathogenesis and immunity. *Vet. Microbiol.* **2013**, *163*, 207–222. [CrossRef]
80. Suankratay, C.; Mold, C.; Zhang, Y.; Lint, T.F.; Gewurz, H. Mechanism of complement-dependent haemolysis via the lectin pathway: Role of the complement regulatory proteins. *Clin. Exp. Immunol.* **1999**, *117*, 442–448. [CrossRef]
81. Sanchez-Larrayoz, A.F.; Elhosseiny, N.M.; Chevrette, M.G.; Fu, Y.; Giunta, P.; Spallanzani, R.G.; Ravi, K.; Pier, G.B.; Lory, S.; Maira-Litran, T. Complexity of Complement Resistance Factors Expressed by Acinetobacter baumannii Needed for Survival in Human Serum. *J. Immunol.* **2017**, *199*, 2803–2814. [CrossRef] [PubMed]
82. Claesson, R.; Kanasi, E.; Johansson, A.; Kalfas, S. A new cleavage site for elastase within the complement component 3. *APMIS* **2010**, *118*, 765–768. [CrossRef] [PubMed]
83. Kanasi, E.; Dogan, B.; Karched, M.; Thay, B.; Oscarsson, J.; Asikainen, S. Lack of serotype antigen in *A. actinomycetemcomitans*. *J. Dent. Res.* **2010**, *89*, 292–296. [CrossRef] [PubMed]
84. Deatherage, B.L.; Cookson, B.T. Membrane vesicle release in bacteria, eukaryotes, and archaea: A conserved yet underappreciated aspect of microbial life. *Infect. Immun.* **2012**, *80*, 1948–1957. [CrossRef] [PubMed]
85. Jan, A.T. Outer Membrane Vesicles (OMVs) of Gram-negative Bacteria: A Perspective Update. *Front. Microbiol.* **2017**, *8*, 1053. [CrossRef] [PubMed]
86. Rompikuntal, P.K.; Thay, B.; Khan, M.K.; Alanko, J.; Penttinen, A.M.; Asikainen, S.; Wai, S.N.; Oscarsson, J. Perinuclear localization of internalized outer membrane vesicles carrying active cytolethal distending toxin from *Aggregatibacter actinomycetemcomitans*. *Infect. Immun.* **2012**, *80*, 31–42. [CrossRef] [PubMed]
87. Demuth, D.R.; James, D.; Kowashi, Y.; Kato, S. Interaction of *Actinobacillus actinomycetemcomitans* outer membrane vesicles with HL60 cells does not require leukotoxin. *Cell Microbiol.* **2003**, *5*, 111–121. [CrossRef] [PubMed]
88. Goulhen, F.; Hafezi, A.; Uitto, V.J.; Hinode, D.; Nakamura, R.; Grenier, D.; Mayrand, D. Subcellular localization and cytotoxic activity of the GroEL-like protein isolated from *Actinobacillus actinomycetemcomitans*. *Infect. Immun.* **1998**, *66*, 5307–5313. [PubMed]
89. Karched, M.; Ihalin, R.; Eneslätt, K.; Zhong, D.; Oscarsson, J.; Wai, S.N.; Chen, C.; Asikainen, S.E. Vesicle-independent extracellular release of a proinflammatory outer membrane lipoprotein in free-soluble form. *BMC Microbiol.* **2008**, *8*, 18. [CrossRef] [PubMed]
90. Kato, S.; Kowashi, Y.; Demuth, D.R. Outer membrane-like vesicles secreted by *Actinobacillus actinomycetemcomitans* are enriched in leukotoxin. *Microb. Pathog.* **2002**, *32*, 1–13. [CrossRef] [PubMed]
91. Kieselbach, T.; Zijnge, V.; Granstrom, E.; Oscarsson, J. Proteomics of *Aggregatibacter actinomycetemcomitans* Outer Membrane Vesicles. *PLoS ONE* **2015**, *10*, e0138591. [CrossRef] [PubMed]
92. Kieselbach, T.; Oscarsson, J. Dataset of the proteome of purified outer membrane vesicles from the human pathogen *Aggregatibacter actinomycetemcomintans*. *Data Brief* **2017**, *10*, 426–431. [CrossRef] [PubMed]
93. Iino, Y.; Hopps, R.M. The bone-resorbing activities in tissue culture of lipopolysaccharides from the bacteria *Actinobacillus actinomycetemcomitans*, *Bacteroides gingivalis* and *Capnocytophaga ochracea* isolated from human mouths. *Arch. Oral Biol.* **1984**, *29*, 59–63. [CrossRef]
94. Ahlstrand, T.; Kovesjoki, L.; Maula, T.; Oscarsson, J.; Ihalin, R. *Aggregatibacter actinomycetemcomitans* LPS binds human interleukin-8. *J. Oral Microbiol.* **2019**, *11*, 1549931. [CrossRef]
95. Choi, J.W.; Kim, S.C.; Hong, S.H.; Lee, H.J. Secretable Small RNAs via Outer Membrane Vesicles in Periodontal Pathogens. *J. Dent. Res.* **2017**, *96*, 458–466. [CrossRef] [PubMed]
96. O'Donoghue, E.J.; Krachler, A.M. Mechanisms of outer membrane vesicle entry into host cells. *Cell Microbiol.* **2016**, *18*, 1508–1517. [CrossRef] [PubMed]
97. Kesty, N.C.; Mason, K.M.; Reedy, M.; Miller, S.E.; Kuehn, M.J. Enterotoxigenic Escherichia coli vesicles target toxin delivery into mammalian cells. *EMBO J.* **2004**, *23*, 4538–4549. [CrossRef] [PubMed]
98. Nice, J.B.; Balashova, N.V.; Kachlany, S.C.; Koufos, E.; Krueger, E.; Lally, E.T.; Brown, A.C. *Aggregatibacter actinomycetemcomitans* Leukotoxin Is Delivered to Host Cells in an LFA-1-Indepdendent Manner When Associated with Outer Membrane Vesicles. *Toxins* **2018**, *10*, 414. [CrossRef] [PubMed]

99. Gholizadeh, P.; Pormohammad, A.; Eslami, H.; Shokouhi, B.; Fakhrzadeh, V.; Kafil, H.S. Oral pathogenesis of *Aggregatibacter actinomycetemcomitans*. *Microb. Pathog.* **2017**, *113*, 303–311. [CrossRef]
100. Hajishengallis, G. Periodontitis: From microbial immune subversion to systemic inflammation. *Nat. Rev. Immunol.* **2015**, *15*, 30–44. [CrossRef]
101. Johansson, A.; Dahlén, G. Bacterial virulence factors that contribute to periodontal pathogenesis. In *Pathogenesis of Periodontal Diseases*; Bostanci, N., Belibasakis, G., Eds.; Springer Nature: Cham, Switzerland, 2018; pp. 31–49. [CrossRef]

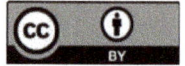

© 2019 by the authors. Licensee MDPI, Basel, Switzerland. This article is an open access article distributed under the terms and conditions of the Creative Commons Attribution (CC BY) license (http://creativecommons.org/licenses/by/4.0/).

MDPI
St. Alban-Anlage 66
4052 Basel
Switzerland
Tel. +41 61 683 77 34
Fax +41 61 302 89 18
www.mdpi.com

Journal of Clinical Medicine Editorial Office
E-mail: jcm@mdpi.com
www.mdpi.com/journal/jcm

www.ingramcontent.com/pod-product-compliance
Lightning Source LLC
LaVergne TN
LVHW070551100526
838202LV00012B/436